CRITICAL ISSUES IN PSYCHIATRY
An Educational Series for Residents and Clinicians

Series Editor: Sherwyn M. Woods, M.D., Ph.D.
University of Southern California School of Medicine
Los Angeles, California

Recent volumes in the series:

CLINICAL DISORDERS OF MEMORY
Aman U. Khan, M.D.

CLINICAL PERSPECTIVES ON THE SUPERVISION OF PSYCHOANALYSIS AND PSYCHOTHERAPY
Edited by Leopold Caligor, Ph.D., Philip M. Bromberg, Ph.D., and James D. Meltzer, Ph.D.

CONTEMPORARY PERSPECTIVES ON PSYCHOTHERAPY WITH LESBIANS AND GAY MEN
Edited by Terry S. Stein, M.D., and Carol J. Cohen, M.D.

DIAGNOSTIC AND LABORATORY TESTING IN PSYCHIATRY
Edited by Mark S. Gold, M.D., and A. L. C. Pottash, M.D.

DRUG AND ALCOHOL ABUSE: A Clinical Guide to Diagnosis and Treatment, Second Edition
Marc A. Schuckit, M.D.

EMERGENCY PSYCHIATRY: Concepts, Methods, and Practices
Edited by Ellen L. Bassuk, M.D., and Ann W. Birk, Ph.D.

ETHNIC PSYCHIATRY
Edited by Charles B. Wilkinson, M.D.

MOOD DISORDERS: Toward a New Psychobiology
Peter C. Whybrow, M.D., Hagop S. Akiskal, M.D., and William T. McKinney, Jr., M.D.

NEUROPSYCHIATRIC FEATURES OF MEDICAL DISORDERS
James W. Jefferson, M.D., and John R. Marshall, M.D.

THE RACE AGAINST TIME: Psychotherapy and Psychoanalysis in the Second Half of Life
Edited by Robert A. Nemiroff, M.D., and Calvin A. Colarusso, M.D.

TREATMENT INTERVENTIONS IN HUMAN SEXUALITY
Edited by Carol C. Nadelson, M.D., and David B. Marcotte, M.D.

A Continuation Order Plan is available for this series. A continuation order will bring delivery of each new volume immediately upon publication. Volumes are billed only upon actual shipment. For further information please contact the publisher.

Ethnic Psychiatry

Ethnic Psychiatry

Edited by

Charles B. Wilkinson, M.D.
Greater Kansas City Mental Health Foundation
and University of Missouri–Kansas City School of Health
Kansas City, Missouri

Plenum Medical Book Company
New York and London

Library of Congress Cataloging in Publication Data

Ethnic psychiatry.

(Critical issues in psychiatry)
Includes bibliographies and index.
1. Minorities, Mental health—United States. 2. Psychiatry, Transcultural—United States. I. Wilkinson, Charles B. II. Title. [DNLM: 1. Ethnic Groups—psychology. 2. Mental Health Services. WA 305 E84]
RC451.5.A2E8 1986 362.2′089 86-8181
ISBN-13: 978-1-4612-9302-6 e-ISBN-13: 978-1-4613-2219-1
DOI: 10.1007/978-1-4613-2219-1

Softcover reprint of the hardcover 1st edition 1986
233 Spring Street, New York, NY 10013

Plenum Medical Book Company is an imprint of Plenum Publishing Corporation

Contributors

ROBIN LADUE, Department of Psychiatry and Behavioral Sciences, University of Washington, Seattle, Washington 98105

CERVANDO MARTINEZ, JR., Department of Psychiatry, The University of Texas Health Science Center at San Antonio, San Antonio, Texas 78284

JEANNE SPURLOCK, American Psychiatric Association, Washington, D.C. 20005

R. DALE WALKER, Seattle Veterans Administration Medical Center, and Department of Psychiatry and Behavioral Sciences, University of Washington, Seattle, Washington 98105

CHARLES B. WILKINSON, The Greater Kansas City Mental Health Foundation, and University of Missouri–Kansas City School of Medicine, Kansas City, Missouri 64108

JOE YAMAMOTO, Neuropsychiatric Institute, University of California Medical School, Los Angeles, California 90024

Foreword

Today there is an overall greater awareness and acceptance of ethnic diversity in American society and a clearer definition of the United States as a pluralistic nation. The last U.S. census showed that well over 100 million Americans, white and non-white, identify with an ethnic group.

Ethnicity is indicative of more than the personal distinctiveness derived from race, religion, national origin, or geography. It denotes the culture of people—that powerful yet subtle factor that shapes values, attitudes, perceptions, needs, modes of expression, patterns of behavior, and identity. From a clinical perspective ethnicity involves conscious and unconscious processes that fulfill deep psychological needs for security, a sense of one's own proper dignity, and a sense of historical continuity as well. These functional aspects of ethnicity reinforce the notion that culture is of significant value to the quality of life and the mental health of all individuals. In the preventive and therapeutic sense, ethnicity sustains a capacity for coping with stress by providing communal support systems which serve to buffer the excessive individualism, alienation, and anomie of modern mass culture. Hence, to ensure appropriate delivery of mental health services to a particular ethnic population, mental health professionals must first become cognizant of the positive aspects and strengths to be drawn from a particular group identity and then incorporate these elements into their treatment strategies or techniques.

This book represents an important initiative in fostering attention to the culture and mental health concerns of Asian/Pacific Americans, blacks, Hispanics, and American Indians. The contributors to this volume are distinguished psychiatrists. They have provided especially astute and sensitive observations of the particular group about whom they have written because they are themselves members of these groups. They offer us insights based on cultural uniqueness that are historically derived.

For many, this book will stimulate awareness of these ethnic cultures, and for others it will augment or reinforce knowledge already gained. For all mental health practitioners, this book provides valuable tools for fine-tuning our approaches to different groups of people in different ethnic circumstances. The fuller understanding of ethnicity that this volume promotes will enhance our capacity to respond to individuals in pain.

Shervert Frazier
Director, National Institute of Mental Health
Rockville, Maryland

Contents

Ethnic Psychiatry

1

Introduction

CHARLES B. WILKINSON

This book is the result of a several-year effort by a selected cadre of professionals with both the breadth of knowledge and the depth of experience in mental issues involving ethnic and minority groups. The book is born out of the recognition of the need in the mental health professions of facts and information pertaining to the disparate life styles, attitudes, and behavior of persons of common ethnic backgrounds and how they are perceived and/or misperceived by others. When care for emotional difficulties is sought, this misperception often results in patients and caregivers being at odds in the mutual establishment of the alliance necessary to provide relief of these problems. So as to shed some light on this frequently encountered dilemma, the authors have attempted to interpret many of the forces that can lead to this kind of patient–therapist impasse and to offer recommendations for the surmounting of these difficulties.

CHARLES B. WILKINSON • The Greater Kansas City Mental Health Foundation, and University of Missouri–Kansas City School of Medicine, Kansas City, Missouri 64108.

Because, in the content of the chapters to follow, several terms that are related but actually have different meanings are used interchangeably, a clarification is in order. Referred to are *ethnicity, social class, race,* and *minorities.* In some instances, all of these terms apply to an ethnic group, while in others, a lesser number defines the group.

ETHNICITY

The word *ethnic* has taken on many different meanings, often representing the idiosyncratic thinking of the user of the term. These meanings may range from the color of skin to birth origin, religious preference, minority group status, class stratification, political affiliation, and even university study programs. An ethnic group is actually "a distinct category of a population in a larger society whose culture is usually different" from that of the larger society.(1) The common bond of an ethnic group may be related to race but can also, or instead, be bound to a common culture or nationality. Depicting groups bound by race is not difficult in this country or, for that matter, in most nations. Understanding conflict between groups with a common race, religious belief, and nationality, however, becomes a little more difficult to explain, e.g., Moslem Sunis and Shiites. There are situations in which ethnic groups share harmoniously the same territory yet maintain differences in language and culture, e.g., some parts of Burma and Thailand. According to Leach,(2) these groups are held together by a traditional system of social relations that is not mandated by a central government. More often, varying degrees of distance and animosity exist between ethnic groups, with power vested in the group(s) with a greater political and economic strength, if not population size.

SOCIAL CLASS AND ETHNICITY

Because "class groups" and ethnic groups may resemble each other behaviorally and culturally, or, for that matter, may be viewed as having similar characteristics, it is important to recognize where differences exist. Sociologists divide society into broad strata that form a hierarchical order of wealth, prestige, and power. In a system of social stratification, individuals belong to a stratum in which they are grouped with like individuals. Each group possesses the following characteristics: All members of the group share ways of acting that are typically different from those in other strata; the group is exclusive and no one can belong to more than one group at the same time; the groups are exhaustive, i.e., everyone in the society belongs to one; and strata are ranked. It has been observed that some small and/or primitive societies with limited populations may not be of sufficient size to be collectivized easily into strata or aggregates of persons of equivalent status. Nevertheless, class status does exist, but group size may not be sufficient to determine clear-cut stratification.(3)

The caste system in India is a form of stratification. The caste groups are not based on ethnicity or on cultural differences but rather are determined by birth. Further, it is a closed system—its members cannot move into another group; groups are maintained because group interrelationships are cooperative rather than competitive.(4) In early studies, South Africa was also viewed as having a caste system; however, the rigid color-bar, with its punitive excesses as a significant aspect of the apartheid, makes it more akin to an estate or plantation system than to any other societal arrangement.(5) In contrast to the rigid caste and estate systems, in some places (e.g., Mexico and parts of the West Indies) ethnic groups are viewed as social classes. Movement from one class to another is permitted. When, however, some of the requirements for membership in a social class are indistinguishable from those for membership in an ethnic category, a structural differentiation between the two is difficult, if not impossible. Those instances in which class and ethnicity coincide make credible the use of the terms interchangeably.

RACE

Race is a major subdivision of mankind, regarded as having a common origin, and is made up of individuals who have a relatively constant combination of physical traits that are handed on from parents to children. Ethnicity and race are often thought of as one and the same, but they do not consistently have the same meaning. *Ethnicity* refers to cultural features while *race* has biological as well as cultural components. Like the word *ethnicity*, *race* is applied in an astonishing variety of contexts and is used to refer to tribes, nation states, language families, and minorities. It has been periodically subjected to intensive scrutiny, has been made the vehicle for justifying racial superiority, and has served as an investigative topic about which many armchair and pseudoscientists have exhibited their ignorance.

Post-Galilean evidence of racism is prominently displayed in Count's account of Carol von Linne's taxonomy of racial characteristics in his *Systems Naturae*, published in 1735.[(6)] In this document a classification of several human varieties was offered. The aboriginal American (American Indian) was described as "reddish in color with straight dense black hair, persevering, content free," and who "paints himself with skillful red lines." Europeans are "light, active, ingenuous, and covered with tailored clothes." Asians were considered "severe, haughty, miserly and covered with loose garments," while

Africans were felt to be "crafty, lazy, negligent, anointed with oil." These racial traits were also regarded as permanent and unchanging. The extent to which many of these descriptions have endured through the years and persevered in the form of racial stereotypes is amazing. Descriptions of this sort proposed a problem for philosophers, scientists, and others who believed in the unitary theory of mankind, for if all men descend from Adam, infraspecies variation somehow had to be explained.(7) Many 18th-century monogenists, however, began to question the permanence of these racial characteristics. Racial differences then began to be considered evanescent and amenable to the control of the natural and cultural forces within the environment.

The doctrine of "perfectibility" of members of the nonwhite race was instead proposed and strongly supported. This was the belief that racial differences would gradually disappear if the causes that produced them were to cease or were somehow altered.(8) This would eventuate in the evolvement of one racial type. Even this more liberal stance reflected a subtle racism since the model was clearly that of the white European. Major supporters of the theory felt that it was possible that negroid physical features were not necessarily hereditary, and in the United States it was argued that dark skin was similar to freckles and that white persons with sufficient exposure to the sun could become negroid. This approached the absurd with the presentation of the reverse of this process in a Virginia slave who lost pigmentation after having moved north. Benjamin Rush, a believer in this theory, argued in 1797 at a meeting of the American Philosophical Society that this proved that black skin color was a disease akin to leprosy.(9) It is unlikely that the move north had any effect on the loss of pigmentation, and vitiligo is still a disease of unknown etiology.

Despite the subtle racist aspects of the doctrine of perfectibility, it did represent an iconoclastic break from the old, overtly racist, theories. It was also open—i.e., it could more readily accept and assimilate new concepts and ideas. Thus, this doctrine had the greater possibility of being modified with the addition of new information. In this regard it was an optimistic, liberal theory that inherently possessed the seeds of egalitarianism.

It is unlikely that the theorists of the doctrine of perfectibility in the 18th century expected the gross modifications that occurred in the 19th century. Increasing insight by scientists into the geological time clock, while continuing the idea of perfectibility, held that Caucasoid man was thousands of years ahead of the other racial groups. Caucasoid characteristics could be acquired but several thousand years might be necessary before equality could be attained. Thus, while the latter remained perfectible, "it effectively removed them from any immediate claim to equal sociopolitical treatment."[(7)] This was of course a very useful theory for the slave-holding states in America and for the European nations that continued economic exploitation of the unfortunate in Asia and Africa who were "less advanced on the evolutionary scale." It provided a ready-made rationalization for the assumption of all sorts of advantages by the "superior races" and atrocities could be subsumed under such philosophies as the white man's burden (slave-holding nations) and the manifest destiny (American Indian). This type of megalomania reached its pinnacle in 20th-century Nazi Germany, culminating in a massive effort at Jewish genocide.

Contributions toward establishing a racial hierarchy were also made by anthropometrists who set about quantifying details of "physiologically insignificant traits" such as the contour of facial and cranial bones as evidence of biological differences.[(10)] The norm against which all other racial groups were compared was naturally Caucasoid. Curiously, even in recent times, differences in racial body structure have taken on brief trivial importance. Questions arose why black track and field athletes excelled in the dashes but not in long-distance competition. A shortened Achilles tendon and other musculoskeletal differences were proposed. These, however, were apparently put to rest in the 1960s as a result of the superior performances by East African athletes in the Olympic distance events.

Much of the credit for debunking racist explanations and separating them from racial groups is credited to the work of Franz Boas and his colleagues.[11,12] It has been subsequently determined that in the relationship between race and culture, the direction of cultural change and the rate with which these changes occur are independent of genetic makeup. If all factors could be kept constant except for race—i.e., if perfect control could be established over enculturation experiences—a single generation is all that would be necessary to equip a member of one racial group with the cultural traits of another. If Zulu babies were substituted for Africander infants, "their average cultural performance would probably not differ in any significant fashion from a control group."[7] Evidence of the susceptibility to cultural influences has been found in virtually every racial group. Indians raised in South America show no resistance hereditarily to learning African dance rhythms, American black vocalists with extensive training perform in operas and concerts in the European tradition, and Japanese who have attained excellence in Western science and technology suffer no hereditary disability from this acquisition. According to Harris,[7] "with the exception of a handful of hereditary pathological disabilities, there does not exist a single instance of differential learning ability between populations which cannot be explained in terms of differential conditioning experience."

MINORITIES

A minority is a group of people who are differentiated from others in the same society by ethnicity, race, nationality, or religion, and who occupy subordinate positions in the communities in which they reside.

A minority group may be numerically smaller but, on the other hand, may constitute the majority insofar as population size is concerned. In several counties in a few southern states, the black population is by far the larger, but in most states and in the United States as a whole, blacks constitute a far smaller percentage of the total population. South Africa and Rhodesia (prior to becoming Zimbabwe) are typical examples of a smaller population group occupying the dominant role in society. In each of the above examples blacks are viewed as the minority group.

The presence of a minority implies that it exists in the presence of a majority. The prototype for the majority in this country is the white Anglo-Saxon Protestant, but considering the size of the innumerable racial and ethnic conglomerates, with almost worldwide representation, this group instead is numerically a minority. It is apparent, then, that designation as a minority relates to something other than the size of the group. According to Rose,[13] a minority position involves assignment to a lesser status and/or exclusion in one or more of four areas of life: economic, political, legal, and social-associational. Exclusion is preserved by the retention of power in the hands of a dominant group. The power is used principally for economic, political, and often sexual exploitation. This is supported by a philosophical belief system attesting to the moral correctness of their stance.

Partial or complete exclusion by the dominant group of the minority group serves to maintain the latter's status as a minority. The minority group tends also to voluntarily exclude itself at least partially from participation in these areas. This is necessary as a collective defense against the harshness and inhumanity of the dominant group; it also serves as a means of maintaining the traditional culture of the group. The nature of the situation breeds hostility, which the dominant group generally has the freedom to express overtly but which must be camouflaged and disguised by the minority group. It is only with the partial lifting of some of the exclusions that the overt hostility of the minority group becomes apparent.

European immigrant minority groups over a period of several generations have been assimilated into the mainstream of American society. However, a loss of the original culture does not necessarily occur following assimilation. The traditional practices may not be a part of everyday behavior but they are evident at the time of important events,—e.g., weddings, births, funeral ceremonies, special holidays. Even if their traditional culture is not considered as an important component of their lives, selected bits of information are passed from generation to generation so that most family members have some knowledge of their original homeland.

The culture of minorities often differs from that of the majority. Even if the original culture is lost, their very exclusion from the general society lays the groundwork for the development of a culture that is deviant from that of the majority.(14) Because of their dissatisfaction with their status in the overall society, minority groups can be source of social unrest. This is particularly so when they form organized groups with the intent of altering the balance of power. This force assumes greater strength when it establishes coalitions with groups within the dominant society. This upsets the *status quo* because it requires the dominant majority to make periodic adjustments in order to accommodate the minority.(13)

America has always been at odds with its national model. The statue in the New York harbor welcomes "your tired, your poor, your huddled masses," yet virtually every minority group has, once on its shores, encountered discrimination. It would perhaps be comfortable for the bureaucracy or the interpreters of the American scene to explain the United States as a melting pot. A true melting pot, however, calls for a relinquishing of those cultures considered alien and would eventually lead to the creation of a homogenized mass. Despite this apparent desire, the United States has not become a melting pot, nor is this likely; rather it is destined to continue as a rich diversity of minorities that constitute its pluralistic society.

GROUP DIFFERENCES AND MENTAL HEALTH

When categorized in any of the aforementioned groups, the respective members are considered different from the dominant group in our society and are treated differently. The combination of their original culture (or remnants thereof) and the developed characteristics resulting from separation tends to set them apart from the dominant majority. These cultural factors pervade every aspect of their behavior and their intragroup and intergroup relationships. Attitudes toward health and mental health reflect these differences. When health providers are of a different group, in order to engage the patient therapeutically, the existing differences must be dealt with appropriately. To understand these alluded-to differences it is important to have some understanding of the historical background and events in the United States of the ethnic groups under consideration. These have been addressed in several of the chapters that follow.

Because of the large numbers of racial and ethnic groups in the United Stated, a choice had to be made for inclusion in this volume. Selected were those groups that for the most part differ physiogonomically from the majority group and toward whom exclusion from the mainstream of America has been practiced and a lower status in society has been assigned.

Thus, American Indians, black Americans, Spanish-speaking peoples, and Orientals and Pacific Islanders constitute the racial and ethnic groups in this book. A critical reader might question if the material here is more referrable to disadvantaged groups in general rather than being ethnic- and/or minority-specific. It is true that most of what is included considers, predominantly, the socially and economically disadvantaged. However, a minority is defined on the basis of its being excluded from the "advantages" held by the majority. It is this exclusion that produces a disadvantaged state. It is also the disadvantaged who to a greater extent maintain their traditional values, since movement into an advantaged category is occasioned by varying degrees of loss of the original culture.

A single volume cannot adequately depict the many issues related to subgroups within each ethnic group. Recognizing this, we have made an attempt—by considering the commonalities where appropriate, and through the history of the experiences of several groups—to provide as complete a picture as is possible. Many of the therapeutic approaches also lend themselves to extrapolation across ethnic groups. Despite the apparent shortcomings, it is the desire and expectation of the authors that this volume can serve as a source of practical information useful to mental health providers and planners in understanding, communicating, and responding to the needs of ethnic group patients requiring help.

REFERENCES

1. H. S. Morris, Ethnic groups, in: *International Encyclopedia of the Social Sciences* (D. L. Sills, ed.), 5:167–172, Macmillan and Free Press, New York, 1968.
2. E. R. Leach, *Political Systems of Highland Burma: A Study of Kachin Social Structure*, Harvard University Press, Boston, 1954.
3. H. S. Morris, The plural society, *Man* 57:124–125, 1957.

4. S. F. Nadel, *The Theory of Social Structure,* Cohen and West, London, Free Press, Glencoe, Illinois, 1957.
5. J. H. Boeke, *Economics and Economic Policy of Dual Societies as Exemplified by Indonesia,* Institute of Pacific Relations, New York, 1953.
6. E. W. Count, This is race: An anthology selected from *International Literature on the Races of Man,* Schuman, New York, 1950.
7. M. Harris, Race, in: *International Encyclopedia of the Social Sciences* (D. L. Sills, ed.), 13:263–267, Macmillan and Free Press, New York, 1968.
8. J. J. Rousseau, *Discours sur l'Origine et ces Fondements de L'inégalieé parmi les Hommes,* Cambridge University Press, London, 1941.
9. T. F. Gossett, *Race: The History of an Idea in America,* Southern Methodist University Press, Dallas, 1963.
10. W. C. Boyd, Has statistics retarded the progress of physical anthropology? *American Journal of Physical Anthropology, New Series* 16:481–484, 1958.
11. F. Boas, *Race Language and Culture,* Macmillan, New York, 1955.
12. F. Boas, *The Mind of Primitive Man,* Free Press, New York, 1965.
13. A. M. Rose, Minorities, in: *International Encyclopedia of the Social Sciences* (D. L. Sills, ed.), Macmillan and Free Press, New York, 1968.
14. G. Allport, *The Nature of Prejudice,* Anchor Books, New York, 1958.

2

The Mental Health of Black Americans

PSYCHIATRIC DIAGNOSIS AND TREATMENT

CHARLES B. WILKINSON AND
JEANNE SPURLOCK

When subjected to prolonged and unjust oppression, people are occupied with two overriding concerns: their physical survival, and the avoidance of, as much as is possible, the attendant psychosocial stress. On a worldwide basis, oppression may be the result of any one of a combination of conditions—e.g., the tyranny of a dictatorship, persecution on the basis of religion, behavior rooted in the belief in ethnic superiority, nationalism, or economic exploitation. For black Americans, the common or universal oppressive condition is racism. When survival in a racist society is less of a threat, however, more attention is directed to psychosocial concerns.

CHARLES B. WILKINSON • The Greater Kansas City Mental Health Foundation, and University of Missouri–Kansas City School of Medicine, Kansas City, Missouri 64108. JEANNE SPURLOCK • American Psychiatric Association, Washington, D.C. 20005.

In recent years, black persons in increasing numbers have sought relief of stress through the mental health system.

Only after the sociopolitical changes and legal events of the 1950s and 1960s did the mental health of blacks become a concern of this country. Prior to that period, the predominant concerns related to control and containment.[1] The snail-paced implementation of the legal mandates described by Clark[2] as carried out "with all deliberate speed" has produced changes but still has left a racist society fundamentally untouched. On the basis of this unchanged societal attitude, it is not unexpected that blacks seeking help for emotional problems would be viewed in a stereotypical way.

Generally, the operational definition of mental illness relates to the failure to adjust to the prevailing concepts of proper behavior.[3] In blacks a variety of now familiar findings are considered evidence of this failure. They range from intergenerational poverty and antisocial behavior to symptoms of mental illness.[4,5] Also, the "failure" of blacks to adjust has almost been dismissed as being the consequence of genetic inferiority, in favor of the more recent theme of maladaptation based on social deprivation.[6,7] The unusual nature of these "abnormalities or peculiar deficiencies" as a result of oppression are thoroughly documented in an abundance of articles found in behavioral science literature.[8,9] A not infrequently held, supposedly liberal theoretical view further concedes that all maladaptive behavioral responses of blacks are both normal and acceptable as necessary for survival and relief of psychosocial stress. This type of theorizing, however, while advocated by some as charitable or generous, maintains for blacks the concept of deficiency and is subtly racist.[1] It further lends pseudoscientific support to the continuation of fixed and ill-formulated paradigms of the black personality and, according to Ellison,[10] establishes a legitimate basis for exercising the traditional way of relating to blacks—i.e., control and containment. From a mental health point of view, these types of concepts influence both diagnostic assessment and therapeutic approaches and contribute to the ignoring of significant content pertaining to individual uniqueness.

DIAGNOSIS, MYTHS, AND STEREOTYPES

The nature of diagnosis dictates, at least in part, the treatment regime. With current advances, particularly as they relate to biological psychiatry, accuracy in assessment is becoming increasingly important, and we are rapidly approaching the time when an incorrect diagnosis followed by incorrect treatment can become life threatening for the patient. Many of the inaccuracies in diagnostic determinations of black patients are due principally to racism and to practices resulting from this disorder, which has produced in many mental health professionals "a myopia as acute as in the most vocal segregationist."[11]

Prudhomme and Musto[11] noted, "Theories of mental illness among Blacks and Whites carried over into the realm of medicine, a double standard similar to that in general society. . . ." Psychiatric diagnosis reflects the societal attitude and its course can be traced historically. The first recorded evidence of this precedent in the United States was noted during the period of slavery, when two psychiatric syndromes specifically related to blacks were advanced. In 1851 a treatise entitled "Diseases Peculiar to the Negro" was published by a Dr. Samuel Cartwright of New Orleans.[12] One of the "illnesses," dysaethesia aethiopica, a euphemism for rascality, caused a slave to perform his duties in a careless, lackadaisical, irresponsible, and headlong manner. The other, drapetomania, was a disease that caused slaves to run away. The possible etiology, according to Cartwright, could have been due to the Negroes' deficiencies in red blood in the lungs.

They were therefore incapable of performing in the same way as whites or of responding to the treatment that was curative for whites. Further, effective remedies for whites could hurt or even kill a Negro.[12] The convenience of these diagnoses in the service of slavery is quite clear.

In postslavery United States:

> When it appeared that the Black had less mental illness, this fact was explained as a natural result of his uncivilized nature . . . interpreted during the nineteenth century as a result of the comforts of slavery or the dull strength of the uncivilized. The turmoil of reconstruction and the subsequent disenfranchisement of the former slave was described as the tumult to which liberty is incident and to which the Black was unable to adjust because of constitutional inferiority."[11]

Thus, the factors causative of mental illness were based on the same reasoning that was applied when it was expedient to account for its reduced incidence.

Abundant examples of the overdiagnosis, underdiagnosis, or misdiagnosis of mental illness in blacks are found in the literature. Cannon and Locke[13] discuss "differential diagnostic patterns for Blacks" and assert that there is a "hesitancy to diagnose Blacks as affectively ill" that is "overly compensated for by a strong tendency to diagnose Blacks as schizophrenic more frequently than Whites." While only limited nationwide statistics concerning diagnosis of mental disorders for blacks are available, it is possible to draw some inferences about possible misdiagnoses from existing data on utilization of psychiatric facilities. For example, admissions to state mental hospitals in 1975 varied dramatically for the four race-sex groups, with alcohol disorders leading among white males at a rate of 79.5 per 100,000 population and schizophrenia among black males at a rate of 197.1 per 100,000. While depressive disorders were the third-ranking diagnosis for white males, this diagnostic category did not even appear among the five leading diagnoses for black males.

Schizophrenia was the leading diagnosis for admissions to state hospitals in 1975 for both white and black females, but once again the race differential was striking. The rate for black female admissions diagnosed with schizophrenia (118.2 per 100,000) was 2.8 times that for white females (42.8 per 100,000). And while depressive disorders ranked second for white females, they ranked fourth for black females.

Although these statistics are confounded by differential facility utilization patterns according to socioeconomic status, they nonetheless reflect biases in the assignment of diagnoses according to race. Such biases are also reflected in local studies. In 1955 Wilson and Lantz[(14)] reported an increase in schizophrenia of black Virginians and attributed this to the gains associated with civil rights actions. Pasamanick[(15)] challenged the validity of the conclusions of this study, pointing to a fall in admissions rates, in the same hospital system, of individuals diagnosed as having manic-depressive psychosis. "When the two rates are summed, the total rate is invariant across the years, from 28.5 per hundred thousand in 1920 to 27.2 in 1955. What has apparently occurred is a change in style of diagnosis rather than an increase in schizophrenia."

Pope and Lipinski[(16)] contend that with all patients there is an overreliance on presenting symptoms alone in determining the presence of schizophrenia, which results in an overdiagnosis of the illness. Other studies point to blacks as being more severely disturbed, resulting in the frequent diagnosis of schizophrenia[(17)]; it is then apparent that in diagnostic assessment blacks are often placed in a position of double jeopardy. It has also been hypothesized that therapists generally tend to view male black clients as withdrawn or aggressive toward others rather than aggressive toward themselves. In addition, the presence of less evident feelings of guilt and less of a tendency to internalize hostility have been attributed to black patients when they are depressed.[(18)] The implication that blacks rarely commit suicide is obvious. Yet figures published in 1971 by the National Center for Health Statistics show that from 1962 to 1967, self-destruction by nonwhite men in their late 20s increased 68% and surged ahead of white men of the same age.[19] It also does not escape notice that depression, in contrast to schizophrenia, is regarded as a more acute illness with a better prognosis.[20]

Age is no barrier for potential bias in diagnosis. At a large eastern mental health center, it was noted that white elderly patients admitted directly with a diagnosis of organic brain syndrome averaged 77.7 years, and those admitted from nursing homes with the same diagnosis were an average of 81.6 years. Elderly black patients diagnosed as suffering from organic brain syndrome were by comparison an average age of 71.7 years.[21] A shorter life-span for blacks may account for this; however, it is also possible that the factors related to the assignment of the more debilitating diagnoses with a poorer prognosis to younger black patients similarly accounts for the earlier diagnosis of organic brain syndrome in elderly blacks.

Black children and families have similarly been the target of diagnostic labels, and it is highly probable, because of the kind of treatment that has been administered, or the lack thereof, that it is in this area that the greater damage to blacks has occurred. The misconceptions established decades ago die a slow death, and even to the present day, vestiges of these myths are still alive. Bender[22] wrote in 1939:

> There has appeared to be a special pattern in behavior disorders of Negro children that displays itself in several ways. This is related to the question of motility and impulse. Two features which almost anyone will concede as characteristic of the race are: (1) the special capacity for laziness and (2) the special ability to dance. The capacity for laziness is the ability to sleep for long periods of time, when it fits the situation. The dancing represents special motility patterns and tendencies.

With an approach to black children embodying these concepts, one shudders to think of the nature of the therapeutic efforts.

For several decades, the black family has been viewed as matriarchal; the "official title," however, was bestowed with the 1965 publication by the Department of Labor on the Negro family.[(23)] Despite protestations by a number of social and behavioral scientists, the belief in the malevolent influence of the black mother on her offspring, particularly the male, remains strong. A great deal of despair is lavished on the offspring of families in which only the mother is present as the family head. Yet this is an area in which some of the more conflicting results (even without regard to ethnicity) have been reported by a multitude of investigators. Several researchers have noted feminine perceptual styles and diminished masculinity in sexual role preference among males.[(24)] At the same time, others have reported excessive masculinity as a compensatory device.[(27,28)] Difficulties in interacting with males and a rejection of femininity have been recorded for females in father absence.[(27,29)] Hunt and Hunt[(30)] describe positive effects for black males but damaging results for white males in the absence of the father from the household.

Investigations by Wilkinson, O'Connor, and Daniels,[(31)] of black single-parent female-headed families reveal that these families are by no means necessarily pathological social units. Not only were the adolescent sons studied by this group noted for the most part to be achievers, but the amount of antisocial activity was minimal. The mothers were determined in their efforts to improve their housing, economic status, and educational opportunities for their children. This was accomplished by the majority of the mothers in the study despite being, or having been on welfare and frequently the head of exceptionally large families.

Rubin,[(32)] in a study designed to test the hypothesis that "Black boys from homes having no adult male figures would have a significantly poorer self image than girls from this type of home, and boys and girls from homes with adult males and females," determined that there was no significant difference. Rubin's conclusion parallels those of Herzog and Lewis[33]: "father absence is only one among an interacting complex of factors which mediate and condition its impact on a growing child . . . even if eventually a significant association can be demonstrated between father absence and one of the adverse effects attributed to it, that impact is dwarfed by other factors of the interacting complex." It also should be noted that fathering is often provided by a male relative or the mother's "significant other." Of equal importance, although seldom acknowledged, is that "the majority of inner city children are in two-parent homes at any given time and a smaller proportion remain in two-parent homes throughout their first 18 years."[33]

In any consideration of causology of emotional illness in blacks, the effects of racism and poverty often become indistinguishable. This is not unusual in that the factors imposed by oppressive racist practices pervade all segments of American society, of which poverty is inevitably one of the results. The paucity of opportunity—economically, in housing, and educationally—collectively leads down a one-way street to poverty. Added to this is the almost daily barrage of insults based solely on race, which has a demoralizing impact on the black psyche. The resultant lowered conception of self-worth, lowered aspirations, and distortion of values in comparison to the view of the societal majority not only affects personality development but also contributes to the maintenance of poverty. Thus, racism and poverty constitute a vicious self-perpetuating cycle, each reinforcing the other.

The destructive impact of these two factors is pointedly described in Mehlinger's[34] report on the evaluation, for a state vocational rehabilitation agency, of 134 prematurely retired black patients in their third and fourth decades of life. He found that the majority had experienced severe poverty and racial oppression, and had suffered extreme social and cultural deprivation. They were generally from large families without the presence of the father, had minimal schooling, and had out of necessity engaged in adult work as early as, in some instances, age 6. Several in their 40s had already worked for as long as the average person does in a lifetime. They were a "washed-out," phlegmatic lot whose overworked psychic defense system had failed, with a subsequent decompensation into frank psychotic manifestations, states of chronic anxiety, or debilitating psychosomatic symptoms. Most were declared unsalvageable.

Despite the breeding ground for potentially devastating psychopathology, a surprising number of blacks manage not only to survive but to surmount these difficulties in the process of achieving varying degrees of success. So while defective ego development is a hazard of the modern ghetto, there is, in managing to survive, also evidence of "resilient strengths which serve to establish effective means of autonomous function in relation to vital task requirements."[35] Society's image of blackness is generally perceived as negative, and although scores of black Americans share this view, which has been reinforced by the findings of some investigators,[36,37] there are many others who have always held themselves in high esteem and see their blackness as a badge of toughness.

A broad range of psychopathological disorders noted in black children are often viewed as characteristically due to racial differences, but their striking prevalence in dismal overcrowded ghetto pockets makes it apparent that poverty is a major factor. Hyperkinesis, pica, learning problems, and unsocialized aggressive reactions of childhood are commonly seen. Poor prenatal care, marred parenting, and the noxious atmosphere of poverty are noted in the history of these families. Despite the fact that the use of lead-free paint is required in most states, lead poisoning must be considered as part of the differential diagnosis of these youngsters when they appear for treatment. The infrequency of the diagnosis of autism leads to reports that this entity is rare in black children, but there is a strong probability that instead of being rare, it frequently may be diagnosed erroneously as mental retardation.

In view of the stress and deprivation that is an integral part of life for many black Americans, it does not appear unusual that there is a high percentage of debilitating mental and physical disorders as well as those related to social deviation. It is, for example, an established fact that across cultural lines, schizophrenia is an illness that is more frequently found in the lower socioeconomic classes.[38,39] Thomas[40] and Comer[41] write of "direct linkages between the quality and level of mental health in individuals and groups and the opportunities and limits that exist within the society." Historical and psychological treatises documenting racism in America abound in the literature and are recorded by a host of authors.[7,40,42–44] They pertain principally to the behavioral dynamics of the oppressors and the direct efforts of racism in the production of a host of psychiatric and nonpsychiatric effects in its victims. However, accurate descriptions of the developmental progression of the dynamic forces that originate in both poverty and racism and result in emotional illness have yet to be articulated.

On the other hand, it is apparent that when mental illness is present, there is less in the way of resources for the poor and the black, and illness is often accompanied by an ignorance and/or an unawareness of how to access those resources that are available. In addition, poverty itself connotes second-class citizenship. Further, the tendency to view black persons from a preconceived stereotypical point of view leads to frequent incorrect diagnosis, followed by indifferent therapeutic considerations. The authors on the one hand protest the overclassification of blacks into certain diagnostic categories and their underclassification into others according to preconceived notions without scientific basis or clinical curiosity as to the origin of symptoms within their contextual frameworks, but they are at the same time acutely aware of the high-risk factors that contribute to these symptom complexes. It is, however, impossible in scanning overall statistics to determine where risk leaves off and misdiagnosis begins.

Much has been made of the difference in symptoms in blacks in comparison to whites. Isolated descriptions of symptomatic differences between black and white patients have been offered to establish a basis for standard diagnoses. Schwab,[(45)] for example, speaks of depression manifested in ambulatory black patients by complaints of headaches that are persistent and of low grade, seldom increase in intensity, and are not relieved by analgesics. Backaches, aches and pains in the extremities, and fatigue complete the picture. Whether this symptom complex clearly differentiates a form of depression in blacks as opposed to nonblacks may have to stand the test of time and continued observation.

There are far more questions in this area of "difference" than there are answers, indicating that there are a number of phenomena pertaining to the black emotionally ill that are fertile grounds for meaningful research. Shader[(46)] suggests the possibility of a different kind of response to psychotropic medication in patients with sickle cell anemia or sickle cell trait because of the state of the red blood cells. The authors also feel that with bipolar illness being diagnosed with increasing frequency in adolescents, there may be a possibility that some hyperactive and destructive black youths may actually belong in this diagnostic category. There may be many other areas indicative of differences between blacks and whites as they relate to symptomatology, genetic uniqueness, and response to treatment. Actual differences in symptoms, however, appear to be related predominantly to life-style rather than to symptom form; i.e., the content of symptoms reflects the life experiences of the patient but the framework of the symptom reflects the universality of the findings that make up a symptom complex.

PROBLEMS RELATED TO TREATMENT

Evidence has been provided by a number of investigators that differential diagnosis and treatment is associated with race. In psychiatric emergency rooms, the type of referral as well as diagnosis varies with the race of the patient. Accuracy in diagnosis appears to depend upon the distance of the sociocultural gap between patient and clinician—the greater the distance, the less accurate the diagnosis and the more nonspecific the disposition.[47] Jackson *et al.*[48] also point out that blacks are seen more often than whites for diagnosis only. Further, whites are more often selected for insight-oriented therapy than blacks, and with greater frequency for long-term psychotherapy.[49] Blacks are also more often seen by paraprofessionals than are whites.[50,51]

In general, black patients receive less-preferred or "second-class" therapy unless their presentation tends to approximate more closely the cultural position of the evaluator. Even when this is the case, some clinicians, because of their own stereotyped thinking born out of long-standing and unchanging prejudices, often cannot believe that blacks can have a similar value system and will assign patients to a therapeutic regime that is inappropriate.

Because of economic status, larger percentages of black than of white patients are seen in public mental health clinics. Even when referred and having made a first visit, blacks are less prone to maintain their contact with treatment facilities.[52] This has been verified by Yamamoto *et al.*[53] and by Sue *et al.*[51] In the latter study, not only did blacks attend fewer sessions than whites, but 52.1% of blacks, in contrast to 29.8% of whites, dropped out after a first session.

Fiman[54] points out, however, that admission rates are not always a good indicator of success because there is a lack of comparable data from private treatment facilities, and further, in public settings the resources that have been established are often based on hypothesized, rather than actual, needs of minority and low-income groups. The latter point may be reinforced by a finding by Warren *et al.*[55] that black families were less satisfied than white with treatment they had received and more negative in their perceptions of clinics and therapists.

In contradistinction to the findings of reduced attendance, a different set of data were recorded by Reddick.[56] In a report of patient addition rates from 261 federally funded community mental health centers, it was found that the other-than-white addition rates were higher in each sex and age category than the white rate. This might be explained on the basis that community mental health centers are both more accessible and more responsive to their catchment area contituents than are the traditional medical centers, general hospitals, and other public clinics. It is also apparent that blacks now associate less stigma with seeking psychiatric care.

The more successful community mental health centers have been those that have adapted to the prevailing cultural values of their catchment area residents. At an inner-city center, Brown[57] noted how futile her attempts were in interpreting late arrival by her black patients or their failure to appear for a therapy hour. They merely acknowledged their lack of promptness but continued to be 15 to 30 minutes late for sessions even when assisted with transportation. Despite an apparent cavalier attitude about time, they nevertheless utilized productively the remaining available time.

As an example of this, Brown described the case of a middle-aged mother of four children, with a severe neurotic depression, who was consistently late for "no reason." Nevertheless, she accepted the therapist as a source of help in the first interview in spite of never before having had psychiatric contact. Despite her tardiness, she utilized her "shortened hour" well and wasted little time in denial of her own role as a factor in her presenting problems. She easily grasped the concept of internalized anger and by the third interview had shed her crippling psychomotor retardation, had a return of appetite, was sleeping better, felt happier, and was devising ways of coping with her innumerable realistic difficulties.

It perhaps could be stated that the patient was enormously resistant and that both her acting-out (lateness) and unwillingness to talk about it was evidence of her successfully keeping the therapist away from her conflictual situation. One might also consider her striking improvement in three sessions to be a transference cure. While the validity of these statements would be difficult to deny, if viewed solely in this vein, two alternatives would probably have been considered—termination or medication with follow-up visits. The therapist chose to attempt psychotherapy, feeling that it was far more important to deal with the patient's problems within the imposed limitations rather than within the context of the therapist's own value system in regard to time.

The way in which people deal with time has been explored by several investigators. Deregowski[58] suggests that concepts related to time differ from society to society, and cross-cultural differences may occur as a result of any one or more of the following: a different attitude toward time, a difference in familiarity with units of time, and a difference in familiarity with numbers. Following a series of investigations, Bartlett[59] concluded that those things that are outstanding and consequently remembered in every group and at every age around a vast variety of topics are, for the most part, the outcome of tendencies, interests, and/or facts that have some societal value stamped on them. Both investigators demonstrate that a different value is placed on temporal phenomena by urban and rural subjects and by primitive and cosmopolitan subjects.

In subcultural groups—e.g., underprivileged blacks—it is probable that the principal factor pertaining to lateness in therapeutic sessions relates to an attitude toward time and the fact that, for them, time has a lesser value attached than it has for middle-class America.[60] For many of them the experience of long hours of waiting in public facilities for medical care has enhanced the lack of concern for being on time for psychiatric appointments. On the other hand, when middle-class blacks show an irreverence for punctuality in psychotherapeutic sessions, the therapist needs to consider if this represents resistance related to therapy or an unconsciously motivated resistance to middle-class values.

Crisis intervention, an old approach that has been rediscovered, has been popularized by the community mental health center movement. For many blacks who make use of public facilities, helpful support may be available at times of severe personal upheaval, but little in the way of follow-up services for looking with any degree of depth into the causes of the crisis is provided. This is more true of general hospital psychiatric clinics than it is of community mental health centers, which are more prepared for this function.

Continuation of treatment of persons who enter only because of a crisis or other immediately troubling symptoms related to anxiety requires a modification of the usual psychotherapeutic approach. A method that is useful is presented in the case exerpt that follows.

R.J. was a 25-year-old noncommissioned officer in his second army enlistment who sought the help of the post psychiatrist because of severe frontal headaches. He was a military policeman and on several occasions had brought prisoners from the stockade to the dispensary for psychiatric evaluation. In conversations with prisoners on the return to the stockade, he had assessed that they had been comfortable with their contacts with the psychiatrist, who was black. He then felt relatively comfortable in making an appointment.

His headaches did not radiate, were constant during working hours, and were more severe when he was least occupied with duty activities. The problem was of approximately 6 weeks' duration and according to him had recently worsened. He recalled the onset shortly after returning by train from Harrisburg, Pennsylvania, where he and another M.P. had taken two prisoners following sentencing. In the exploratory interview he detailed, at the therapist's direction, events before and after this trip. Further, there was no evidence of an aura, gastrointestinal difficulties, spread of the pain to any other part of the head, or a family history of headaches, epilepsy, or similar disorder. He was a high school graduate who had held an unskilled laboring job for a year prior to his first hitch in the army.

He was noted to be a rather passive, gullible young man, who responded principally to questions with little or no elaboration. Once-weekly interviews were arranged, but he soon fell silent, waiting for the therapist to provide direction. It was apparent that silence provoked only more anxiety but no additional responses. His headaches meanwhile remained unchanged. On the fourth visit, hypnosis was suggested, and the therapist provided him with a full explanation in order to relieve him of any feelings of its being a mysterious and/or frightening procedure. He accepted this, and on the fifth visit hypnotic sessions began. He was a good subject and entered a trance quite easily. Under hypnosis, he related that on the day before his train trip, he sat with his girlfriend, a WAC, in the enlisted men's club and she commented on a pimple on his nose and proceeded to squeeze it. He thought no more of the incident, and while preparing to leave Harrisburg two days later, he stopped to purchase several magazines to read on the trip back to his duty station. While lying in his bunk, he read an article relating to possible spread of infections from the facial area to the brain, and that the picking and squeezing of facial pimples should be avoided. The therapist questioned a possible connection between these events and his headaches, and the soldier was able to grasp this. The unlikelihod of a vascular-borne infection from the face to the brain, as over a month had passed since the incident, was pointed out to him. He was then told that he could recall as much of the session posthypnotically as he wished. After awakening he was asked what he could remember while hypnotized. He had almost total recall of the hypnotic exchange, including the correction of his concerns about a brain infection following the squeezing of the pimple by his girlfriend. Before leaving, the soldier reported a lessening of his headache.

During the next two visits, R.J. was completely free of headaches and was unproductive but denied that he wanted to terminate. He acceded to being hypnotized again on his seventh visit and was able to relate that he wanted to bring his visits to a halt but felt that he could not comfortably state this to an officer and superior. He was told clearly that indeed he could indicate that he wished to terminate and had no need to fear reprisal. Again the soldier was told that he could recall as much as he wished upon awakening. Before the hour ended, although he did not recount what was remembered under hypnosis, he was able to state that he wanted to terminate his sessions. The therapist agreed and also made it clear that he could return if he again felt the need.

R.J. requested an appointment 2 months later, stating that his headaches had returned. They were similar to what he had experienced before and were of 1 week's duration. His story was not unusual, but it became apparent that he was having problems with both his sergeant and his girlfriend. Upon inquiry, he provided more details of these situations, but it was apparent that major sections were being omitted.

Hypnosis was again begun with the second session. Over the course of two visits a week apart, it was gradually revealed that both his first sergeant and his commanding officer were pushing him for reenlistment. His WAC girlfriend, on the other hand, was insisting upon marriage and their leaving the army together. He felt unable to deal with the situation and was uncertain about what to do. While he did not wish to marry at this time and wanted to pursue a career in the military, he was puzzled about her considering their relationship so seriously and also felt guilty in that he might have misled her. Interviews were handled as before; i.e., he was told while hypnotized that he could recall as much as he wanted and that an exchange would take place after the trance. He was able over four sessions to recognize his efforts to escape dealing with his situation and ultimately worked it out with his girlfriend. His headaches began gradually abating during this time. He terminated abruptly when, as a part of his reenlistment, he was transferred to another post.

This young man's dependency and passivity are immediately apparent. It is evident that he thrives when directed by authority, accounting for his desire to remain in the military. As often as possible conflictual situations were avoided by him, as were independently made decisions. When these were inescapable, he demonstrated that he tended to somatize. It is probable that the somatic pathway for his anxiety had been reinforced by the first incident that brought him in to see the therapist.

Considering these factors, one could be inclined to delve further into the "mysteries" of his characterology. Dependency, however, was such a strong factor that regressive material would only serve to intensify his needs. This brings up the issue of hypnosis, which could serve in the same cause; the therapist, however, attempted to reduce this risk by first providing a full disclosure of what hypnosis was about and also by making him responsible at a conscious level for the material talked about while under hypnosis. Further, the focus was maintained on immediate conflict situations.

The periodic therapeutic contacts likely would have continued in the same way had the patient not transferred to another post. This interrupted therapy or "piecemeal" approach to working with patients can conceivably result either in dealing with enough of the major conflicts to eventually leave the patient relatively symptom-free or, occasionally, in the patient's entering therapy on a more consistent basis.

In black patients, particularly those entering public facilities, immediate threats of a crisis or near-crisis are often the cause of their seeking therapy, and after relief of these pressures there is frequently a reduction or dropping off of motivation.

In dealing with this pattern, Sager *et al.*[61] formalized the aforementioned interrupted or piecemeal approach for individual patients and families from ghetto settings. After successfully helping the patient and/or the family deal with the presenting crisis in a limited number of sessions (10 to 15), the therapist then encouraged them to terminate. A number returned because of another crisis, often precipitated when new responsibilities were assumed. Generally, they worked toward achieving further changes that were not considered during the first group of sessions. It has been the author's experience that if attempts are made to retain many of these patients in treatment, there is little or no drive toward doing further work since their own mission or purpose has been accomplished, and subsequent scheduled visits, unless there is another crisis, are occasioned by periods of tense silence, lateness in arrival for the appointed hour, absenteeism, or dropping out of therapy.

The type of therapeutic approach and its subsequent effectiveness is dependent upon the therapist's assessment of the patient. An accurate evaluation of the psychological status of an individual can be made only in relationship to what is considered appropriate and effective functioning within that individual's own specific cultural milieu.[(62)] If this is not kept in mind, then the frequently noted differences between patient and therapist of social, economic, and/or cultural status will lead to the erroneous practice, on the part of the latter, of using his or her own status as the norm and that of the patient, if different, as the deviation from the norm.

Two case reports by Bradshaw,[(63)] representing two extremes in character makeup and symptomatic presentation, demonstrate these early misperceptions.

A.D. was, when seen by the examiner, a 30-year-old black unmarried mother of two children with complaints of pains in the head, neck, and upper and lower back. Her complaints followed being struck on the head at her job at the local post office and were of 2 years' duration. She was examined by a neurosurgeon but there were no pathological findings. For her pain, physical therapy was prescribed and was increased in frequency when after 2 weeks her pain worsened. When this treatment proved ineffective, a cervical myelogram was done which also was negative but was followed by an intensification of pain and several episodes of fainting. Finally, the neurosurgeon recommended that she see a psychiatrist, which she readily accepted because her symptoms had already caused her to cease working and also interfered with her ability to take care of her family.

The psychiatrist was a psychodynamically oriented young white male who, after taking a history, saw her for 10 visits but without improvement. Workman's Compensation refused to pay for her additional visits, so her treatment came to a halt. In a written report, her psychiatrist formulated that her hysterical neurosis was related to difficulties she had in expressing aggression and conflicts over dependency needs. She was considered resistant and would require more time for therapeutic results.

The patient became increasingly depressed over her debilitation and inability to work and sought help at a community mental health center. At the center she was seen by an older white psychiatrist who took a direct approach with her. He prescribed Valium and Mellaril and gave her 15-minute appointments every 2 weeks. When he reduced her treatment time to 10 minutes and decreased the frequency to once monthly, she ceased attending. This psychiatrist's written report indicated that she was of below-average intelligence and not "psychological minded."

The above treatments covered a period of approximately a year. Almost a year following her last psychiatric contact, she managed with legal assistance to have her compensation case reopened. She was again referred to a psychiatrist, this time to the reporter, to whom the earlier psychiatric reports were made available.

The patient was one of eight children and from a rural background. She managed to complete high school; a year later her mother died, and shortly afterwards she became pregnant with her first child. She came to the city at age 21 with her son and worked successively as a domestic, a secretary, and finally a postal service employee. Ms. D. also has had difficulty either in finding or being attracted to men who were reliable and truly interested in her.

When an inquiry was made of her previous psychiatric contacts, she was surprised that she was invited to express her opinions. She stated that her first psychiatrist was well intentioned and interested but that most of the time "we just sat and looked at each other without saying a word." About her second psychiatrist, she felt that he was not interested in her and only wanted to give her medication, which made her sleepy.

Her attention was then directed to her personal life at or about the time of her work accident, and her conditions and/or interpersonal relationships at work. In regard to the former, the patient related that just 2 weeks prior to her accident she had asked the man with whom she had lived for a year to leave because "He was willing to eat my food and sleep in my bed but he wouldn't contribute nothing for the food and rent and he wouldn't be good to my kids." On her job she had experienced increased stress with a new supervisor who was demanding and petty.

DOCTOR: "I'll bet you're the kind of person who doesn't show her feelings directly, particularly when you're annoyed."
PATIENT: (Smiling) "I almost never show my feelings."
DOCTOR: "Even when you want to explode."
PATIENT: "Sometimes I feel like just screaming and hitting people."
DOCTOR: "Like the boyfriend you kicked out, and your supervisor?"
PATIENT: "Yes! Yes!"

By the time of the second session, the patient was almost symptom-free. Her case was accepted for compensation on the grounds that her difficulty was precipitated by the work accident. Since the evaluating psychiatrist could not continue with her, Ms. D. was referred to another therapist. The latter reported that she continued in treatment, remained asymptomatic, returned to work, and made progressive gains in attaining insight in regard to her thinking, feeling, and behavior.

Few responses on the part of the patients considered chronically ill are as dramatic as this. Ms. D. is an unsophisticated, passive young black female for whom life held few pleasures but much in the way of responsibilities and hard work. She had little expectation of further improving her lot in life, and the thought that she might have control over her own destiny had probably never occurred to her. While there is insufficient evidence from only two contacts to support the fact that she set herself up to be taken advantage of by men, it can be assumed that this is correct, and it is apparent that she has been victimized repeatedly. Considering her seeming passivity and reticence in giving vent to her feelings, one has to admire her perspicacity; this unworldly woman sensed that relief should come through psychiatric contacts and managed, despite failures, to continue to seek treatment.

Her first psychiatrist's approach, successful with educated, sophisticated patients, was completely out of place with her. She, however, recognized her therapist's interest in her but did not know what she was supposed to do or how therapy worked. She therefore could not understand his silence, and he made no attempt to explore hers. She held her physicians in awe, which made it even more difficult to be spontaneous. Because he represented, to her, respected authority, she would have naively followed his directions had he given her any. Low-income patients, accustomed to being directed by authority figures, may become bewildered or frightened by a nondirective approach.[41]

The second psychiatrist's handling of her represents the epitome of what should not be done. It is evident that he made certain assumptions when she entered; i.e., she was incapable of profiting from the "talking kind of treatment," and the only approach considered useful involved the use of medication. Follow-up contacts were solely to determine her response to medication and to check for possible side effects. The patient rightfully sensed his disinterest and dropped out. His written report summed up his attitude and preconceived notions of how this type of patient should be handled. His statements "below average intelligence" and "not psychological minded" embody an expressed opinion sans history, sans assessment.

She could not believe that anyone, particularly a man, could really be interested in what she was feeling or thinking but, once given the opportunity, very quickly began to grasp the tenets of therapy.

> The second case is that of J.E., a 28-year-old black male referred to the psychiatric outpatient clinic of a university medical center. He was seen originally in the neurology clinic, but after several verbal altercations with a black neurologist, the patient was told that he would not be permitted to return unless he simultaneously sought psychiatric care. Mr. E. was being treated with nerve stimulation as a part of his rehabilitation for chronic pain in his right arm, secondary to having been shot in the brachial plexus. His injury occurred 4 years earlier when, as a part of a gang, he was caught in a bank robbery. The patient turned state's evidence and was given a short sentence. He suffered severe pain in the arm from the time of the injury and after release attended the pain clinic at a prestigious university hospital in another city. His treatment covered a period of a year and a half and was not successful. A lengthy treatment sum-

mary forwarded from the pain clinic detailed his neurological and muscular limitations and the variety of treatment measures used. The report further indicated that attempts at psychological assistance with individual and group counseling produced limited results, due to "secondary gain and the patient's sociopathic personality."

In the present clinic, the patient was first seen by a black male medical student rotating on a clerkship. The student's negative impression was evident from his chart recording of the description of the patient's swagger, and his "superfly" appearance—i.e., his broad-brim hat, sunglasses, neck chains, open shirt, and platform shoes. The student's unabashed dislike of the patient was further apparent in his diagnostic impression of malingering. At the third interview, the student challenged the patient directly about his alleged inability to work because of pain. This provoked an angry verbal outburst from the patient, and the interchange between the two had to be interrupted by a social worker. It was decided that the student should not continue seeing the patient, who was then assigned to a psychiatric resident.

The patient's chart was reviewed by the resident and a supervisor prior to the first interview. The supervisor did not feel that he was a promising psychotherapeutic candidate but indicated that perhaps something could be learned by obtaining a comprehensive history. He further reminded the resident that the behavior of the patient had aroused negative feelings in everyone who had seen him, which was important to attempt to understand.

The resident was a low-key, calm, somewhat matronly and accepting young black woman. Her overall appearance and manner were nonthreatening.

Over a half dozen sessions, the following historical data emerged. The patient's father left the home when the patient was age 6. On the few times that he saw the patient, he would "put him down," call him a sissy, etc.

Mr. E. felt he could never live up to this cruel man's expectations. By his own admission he was close to his mother; only when he reached adolescence did he find a modicum of male self-esteem and this was principally through athletic activities. When he was 15 he attempted to stand his ground during one of his father's tirades and was beaten rather severely by him. He recalls his father saying, "You're nothing but a punk and that's all you'll ever be." He shortly thereafter dropped out of school, held a succession of jobs, and became a ne'er-do-well. Although growing up in a tough neighborhood, he remained on the fringe of antisocial activity, involved occasionally in minor shoplifting.

Mr. E. married at 21 and began working in a grocery store. After the birth of their first child he began to become painfully aware of his limitations—e.g., education, employability—and felt ill-equipped to provide "the good life" for his family. He then started dressing flashily and hanging out with a "more hip group." Although he was apprehensive about the bank robbery when it was proposed by his friends, the temptation of "making a big score" and proving his manhood by sticking it out with his criminal associates sustained his motivation. Ever the loser, he was the only one of the group who was shot and apprehended on the scene.

The patient is pleased with the image he projects, and secretly exults in the fear that he strikes in others. On the other hand, he is exquisitely sensitive to the slightest implication of a put-down, making him somewhat testy with males in authority. His flamboyance is also accentuated when he wishes to impress a woman: "I present an image of health and wealth."

The resident elicited these data by steering a gingerly course between careful respect for his narcissistic sensitivity and exploration of the defensive function of his external behavior and appearance—e.g., "It seems that it is very important to you that you affect people in a certain way . . . do you have any ideas why creating that image is so important?"

Within a short time, the patient was able to talk about his wounded sense of masculinity. Whenever the facade evaporated even briefly, it was noted that he unconsciously stroked and caressed his injured arm. This was even more striking when he volunteered, with a great deal of difficulty and hesitation, that he was frequently impotent.

After several months of therapy, Mr. E. began to gain some understanding of his compensatory demeanor; continued improvement occurred during intensive, insight-oriented twice-weekly psychotherapy.

It is apparent that the patient's threatening, "supermasculine" behavior was a long-standing defense for his inadequate male identification and a denial of his passive feminine strivings. His ability to create discomfort and fear in potential caregivers served well in reinforcing his defense and in lending evidence to his feeling of superiority over others, despite its ego-alien nature. This behavior consistently provoked sexual and aggressive countertransference feelings in his would-be helpers. With the weakening of his facade, he became symptomatic, revealing at the same time the conversion nature of his difficulty.

Despite his efforts at obtaining acceptance from his father, there was consistent rejection by this cold, cruel parent. He attached himself to his mother in his early years and never actually successfully negotiated his oedipal period.

Considering his behavior, it is not unusual that psychopathy would be diagnosed, and both black and white helping professionals were "taken in" by his presentation. The acceptance of his diagnosis results in an overlooking of the attendant implications regarding ego and superego structure and treatment potential. Perhaps the only initial clue that would allow one to question such an assumption is his persistence in seeking help, which he managed to do while at the same time pushing away and intimidating the very persons from whom he sought relief. That this assumption was premature is evidenced by his response to an accepting therapist who remained unperturbed by his behavior.

Both of the above patients required not only attention to countertransference and cultural differences but also a level of technical skill found infrequently in settings where lower-class blacks are apt to be receiving psychiatric assistance.

When the treatment of the black patients is considered, the preponderance of literature deals almost exclusively with the poor black—the disadvantaged ghetto black. Little attention is paid to the burgeoning black middle class with its own set of problems. Upwardly mobile blacks tend to take on the attitudes, aspirations, and desires of the major pacesetters, the white middle class. There are differences in values and life-styles between middle-class and lower-class blacks just as there are differences between middle- and lower-class whites.[64]

Over the past two decades a wide range of employment opportunities have opened up to blacks, allowing those who avail themselves of them to achieve an economic and social status that was heretofore unavailable. The attainment of these gains is accompanied, however, by an increase in responsibility, and many blacks, unprepared for this different kind of setting or unable to adapt quickly, respond with a variety of symptoms related to stress. Despite an often auspicious start, anxiety mounts when job-related obligations intensify. This is particularly true when the black employee is from a background in which the major decisions in life are attached primarily to supporting immediate needs and perhaps a relatively few luxuries. A request for help or an admission of discomfort is akin to an acceptance of ineptness and is perceived as a blow to the self-concept. The attendant anxiety may be defended against by increasing indifference, a display of incompetence and ineffectiveness not in keeping with actual ability, avoidance of responsibility, absenteeism, and alcoholism. Racial situations may be magnified and used as the *raison d'etre* for job difficulties. If the patient is married, a gamut of family problems may be noted that reflect both individual psychopathology and those symptoms that are a "fallout" from intrafamilial conflicts involving principally the spouse but also the children.

A review of 10 young black married couples who sought treatment during a 2-year period reveals a number of the aforementioned problems and symptoms.[65] These couples were seen conjointly for at least part of their treatment. They ranged in age from 25 (husband) and 23 (wife) to 39 (husband) and 36 (wife), with family incomes ranging from a low of $20,000 to a high of $40,000. All of the males with the exception of two were in managerial or supervisory positions, and one was self-employed. All of the females worked, only three did not function in a managerial or supervisory capacity, and one had an independent income as well. All of the families had children, the smallest number being one (in four couples); in the largest family, there were six children.

In all of the families, it was the wives (of whom five were themselves symptomatic) who initiated the visit to a therapist. In two, it was the husband's complaints that caused help to be sought, and in the remaining three, the problems were because of the children, due usually to acting-out behavior. In one instance, a husband and an only child were symptomatic. Alcoholism on the part of the husband in two instances, and of the wife in a single instance, compounded the family problems.

All but one member (a wife) of the 10 couples completed high school and two husbands attended college, but there were only three college graduates in the entire group, all of whom were wives. Review of the socioeconomic status of the couples' primary families reveals that four of the wives came from families that ranked higher than the husband on the socioeconomic scale; in two instances the husband's family was higher, and in four they were approximately the same—i.e., both husband and wife were from the lower socioeconomic stratum.

In determining which of the spouses were the dominant figures, it was noted that the wives were in seven of the families. In six of these instances, the wife also earned the higher salary; this differential in two of the families was as much as $3,500. These wives were frequently dissatisfied with their husbands' apparent lack of ambition and often openly critical of the seemingly slow, plodding progress in their employment.

The husbands were generally capable and hardworking, but four admitted discomfort in their lower management roles and one became symptomatic after promotion. Two expressed feelings of being held back because of race, one of whom was found to be somewhat paranoid. Their job-related tension was occasioned by frequent absences from work (two) and alcoholism (one). Those whose wives were noted to be particularly aggressive overtly exhibited varying degrees of dependency and passivity and were resentful of their wives' nagging domination, show of superiority, and expensive tastes.

The ending was not happy for these families. Of the 10, 3 divorced, but in one family each ex-marital partner continued treatment individually; divorce was imminent in 1 at the time of this writing, although they also remained in treatment. Four families remained intact and continued in conjoint therapy but the relationships were tenuous. One family dropped out of treatment, and in another, two of the children were in therapy.

These 10 families demonstrate some of the difficulties that

occur in young blacks who exert themselves in order to share the benefits of America through employment opportunities closed to their forebears. The findings they exhibit are not unlike those of many nonblack families in a state of change, although the authors are aware that a respectable number of blacks make the transition with less overt difficulty. On the other hand, it is likely that these findings are seen in greater frequency in black families in which one or both spouses are first-generation upwardly mobile.

A number of findings appear to confirm this probability. Evidence strongly indicates that social mobility is significantly related to emotional disorders and disturbances in interpersonal relations. Rates of illness are higher for both the upwardly mobile and the downwardly mobile than for the socially stable or nonmobile population.[66–69] It has been found that as the distance moved (either upward or downward) increases, the rate of illness also increases.[70] Social climbers particularly have been found to be more subject to chronic psychosomatic disorders.[71]

Not too dissimilar findings of a psychosomatic nature were reported in a study by Holmes,[72] in which tuberculosis morbidity rates were correlated with four Seattle, Washington, census tract-designated residential areas (index of lifestyle): city's center (skid row), blue-collar, white-collar, and better socioeconomic area. Whites in the city's center showed a high morbidity rate, which decreased progressively in the other three areas. The nonwhite rate in the city's center, however, was even higher than the white rate, but only one-half as high in the blue-collar and white-collar areas. The nonwhite rate for morbidity, however, in the better socioeconomic area was one-third again higher than that of the city's center nonwhite group. Holmes[72] postulates that the cultural conflict engendered by close residential juxtaposition of a minority and majority population may evoke depression, withdrawal, and feelings of being overwhelmed, thereby reducing resistance to infection.

In the 10 black families, psychosomatic illness was not a presenting factor, nor was the location of their housing as much of a problem as was their change in employment status. Durkheim's[73] concept of anomie* might better illustrate the sociopsychological aspects of their plight. He maintained that the structure of human nature made the individual's needs and desires insatiable if not restrained by an external regulatory force. The significant social groupings to which the individual belongs is the regulatory body and provides consensus pertaining to the range of legitimate striving (aspirations). When this force is disrupted or shattered, the individual experiences anomie. Status transition disrupts the individual's integration with his social group and weakens the restraints on the individual's aspirations. It is probable that blacks finding themselves for the first time in the position of a status change may experience a lowering of self-esteem, ambivalence in their ethnic identification, and a devaluation of their own accomplishments in comparison to others, all of which makes them vulnerable to problems in interpersonal relationships and psychiatric and psychosomatic disorders. Further credence to Holmes's[72] theoretical assumptions is

* Merton, as quoted in Kleiner and Dalgard,[70] takes a different view of anomie, but his hypothesis would appear to explain the disparaging position of lower-class blacks rather than those attempting to elevate their status. He defines anomie as the "disjunction between means–ends relations" in society; i.e., society through one's own reference group socializes the individual to aspire to specific goals. If the opportunities for realizing these goals are closed or inaccessible due to social barriers, the individual is functioning within an anomic situation. If then, "the Black lower class culture fosters the belief that the opportunity system is closed, then the motivational characteristics of lower class individuals will not include the traditional middle class emphasis on the success ethic, their self esteem will be intact; the risk of mental illness will be low and the risk of delinquency high."

provided by evidence from several studies suggesting that good mental health can serve to extend good physical health. The converse appears also to be true; i.e., poor mental health increases susceptibility to organic diseases.

FOLK MEDICINE HEALING

For a small fraction of blacks with problems, sources other than the helping professions are found, and those believers in folk medicine or hexing are the least likely to seek or accept psychiatric intervention. Instead, folk healers or spiritualists are sought. The use of such healers appears to be dependent on the prevailing culture. In years past, this predominantly existed in rural areas, but with migration to larger urban areas, many persons have brought their beliefs with them, resulting in their dispersal in the overall black population. The principal characters in black folk medicine in ascending order of importance are described by Jordan.[43]

The "Old Lady" (also Granny or Mrs. Markus) is usually knowledgeable in the use of herbs and deals generally with common ailments. Principally, she provides advice and instruction, but she also gives medication. Her assistance is sought most often by young mothers who feel a need for help in raising their infants or in dealing with illness of their young offspring.

The "spiritualist" is the most frequently found folk healer and is "called" to the practice. The subjects treated by the spiritualist, according to Jordan,[43] are described as often fearful and phobic. The spiritualist helps them to better manage their daily lives, sometimes conducting a "practice" via the mails.

The older and most powerful of the group is the voodoo priest or *hougan*, whose training is formalized. Most users of his services are found in the southeastern part of the United States. The priest is noted to be well acquainted with the habits and sicknesses of animals and bases much of his diagnosis and treatment abilities on their self-selection of plant life for healing purposes. Symbolic characterization of animal life is also important, and ingestion of certain organs or parts of specific animals is prescribed in correcting deficiencies. The priest is said to be well oriented in the skills of dealing with individual and family personal problems.

SPECIAL PROBLEMS RELATED TO THE TREATMENT OF BLACK PATIENTS

Therapy philosophically based in intrapsychic dynamics usually relates directly or indirectly to psychoanalytic concepts. Up to a decade or so following World War II, it was believed that blacks were unsuited for, and could not profit from, psychoanalysis or psychoanalytic approaches. With modifications of classical techniques, particularly in this country, this belief has been for the most part nullified, and there is little in psychoanalytic-oriented therapy that is useful for all patients that is not applicable for blacks. In situations in which basic life needs are foremost, however, the therapist may have to resort to pragmatic expediency before conducting what we regard familiarly as therapy. Nevertheless, his knowledge of internal dynamics, if not too rigidly applied, will be useful in understanding his patients.

As with all patients, the most pressing concerns are those with which they must currently deal. For the poor black ghetto dwellers these more often pertain to the most concrete of things such as finding employment; surviving on a welfare budget; seeking housing outside a rat-infested, crime-ridden neighborhood; and/or obtaining clothing so that children can attend school. Whether the therapist working with such patients is active personally or whether he assigns the task of relieving these problems is unimportant as long as he is involved. Active assistance in attempting to lessen the patient's overwhelming burdens should not be viewed as merely a prelude to, or a means of, induction into the "real treatment" but rather as an integral and essential part of the treatment itself.[(61)] Only after dealing with these crisis-provoking situations can the patient and the therapist begin to contend with damaging underlying psychological factors.

There is some opinion that because of the commonality of race and experience, black therapists work better with black patients, but it is unrealistic to expect that black therapists in sufficient numbers will ever be available to provide such services. Necessarily, a large number of black patients will be seen by other than black therapists.

In long-term approaches to psychotherapy, two significant factors are paramount: (1) It is crucial that the therapist make every effort to know and understand the patient's cultural patterns and value systems,* and (2) he must examine his own attitudes, beliefs, and feelings as they arise in conjunction with his work with patients.[(74)]

For the white therapist working with white middle-class patients, the first of these factors, due to a similarity in backgrounds and value systems, can be negotiated more easily. It is when differences exist—e.g., race, sex, age, or economic

* A word of caution is extended by Waite,[(74)] who warns of two potential dangers associated with too active an interest in cultural aspects of the ethnic group of the patient in treatment. He holds that an investment of the psychological energies in this kind of interest tends to allow the therapist to avoid facing his own anxiety at times of conflictual situations and thus operates in the service of countertransference resistances. A second danger relates to the therapist's utilizing his overidentification with the uniqueness of the individual to generalize for all members of the particular minority group.

class—that difficulties may be encountered. For the white therapist from an American background of a 300-year history of discrimination and racial segregation, there is a repository of outstanding myths about black persons that serve to provide him with readily available preconceptions. The more prevalent myths have been classified into seven categories by Bradshaw.(75)

1. Africans arriving in the United States as slaves were of "primitive stock"; they had no culture or civilization of their own.
2. The black family is a tangle of pathology as opposed to the white nuclear family.
3. A matriarchal structure is universal in black families.
4. The black family is in total disarray because of slavery.
5. Psychopathology is the inevitable consequence of one-parent families; strengths cannot emanate from such families.
6. The black man is totally inferior sexually or, conversely, he is a "superstud."
7. Blacks rarely develop severe depressions or commit suicide.

To these may be added, "Blacks are emotional and impulsive, think only concretely, and cannot grasp abstract ideas."

These myths, or some form of them, may be consciously or unconsciously a part of the prospective therapist's thinking at the time of the first encounter with a black patient. He may find the presentation of silence and apparent passivity in a black patient to be frustrating; similarly, he may find "jive talk" and a swaggering, aggressive manner to be intimidating. These can serve to reinforce the therapist's existing stereotypes. Even when they are not a part of conscious thinking of whites, there may be a shocking revelation when a particular type of behavior on the part of the patient reactivates an old, deeply ingrained racial prejudice, long denied and thought to be ego-alien.

With the separation of the races and an environment that supports myths and stereotypes about anyone different from one's self, it can only be expected that the white therapist brings with him to the therapeutic situation varying degrees of misconception. This is why self-examination is of the utmost importance.

Black therapists are not necessarily immune to these same reactions. The effort necessary to become a professional places them in a middle-class category. Coupled with the fact that most blacks receive their psychiatric training in white institutions, their own identification with whites and white middle-class values can prompt a denial of identification with the race of their black patients.

The black patient also has his own stereotypes, and he does not leave them at home simply because he is seeking help. The white therapist is viewed as are whites in general—i.e., as disinterested, dishonest, quick to show "superiority" or to be patronizing and condescending—all of which leads to some gain on the part of the latter at the expense of the patient. He is therefore cautious and wary lest he unexpectedly again be taken advantage of, or subjected to a put-down. With better educated patients these feelings may be hidden, or even denied, behind a facade of sophistication. When the black patient encounters a black therapist who is a part of an institutional setting, the therapist may be viewed as a part of the "oppressive system" and is related to with the same degree of caution or suspicion as is the white therapist.

Some black patients "play dumb" in the presence of white persons—e.g., passive, outwardly compliant, pleasant, and monosyllabic. This is frequently a coping device that has been a necessary accommodation for survival in an alien world, but it is not adaptive when in treatment. The therapist, in working with this type of patient, must assume an active supportive position in order to establish rapport. If the patient's stance is taken at face value, the therapist may bring about premature closure of treatment. Even more destructive for the patient are those instances in which the therapist's preconceived notions include the belief that black patients are inarticulate and unintelligent and therefore unsuitable for psychodynamic therapy. The response of the patient in these instances is predictable, and he may oblige the therapist by simply dropping out of treatment.

To embark on a therapeutic course, a meaningful relationship will have to develop. The same tenets of any therapeutic relationship apply here: respect, interest, and empathy. In some situations with black patients the means by which this is accomplished may necessitate a departure from the classical means of conducting psychotherapy (as was noted earlier with the poor black ghetto dweller).

When working with someone of a different race, some therapists feel it is important that in the initial contact an inquiry be made into the patient's feelings about the arrangement. It is felt that the boldness of such an approach challenges the patient to deal with his own prejudgments. It also indicates the degree to which the therapist is open to such matters.[(76)] (Exceptions to this are brief or emergency—crisis—encounters. But even in such instances if racial differences interfere with aiding the patient, the subject should be introduced.) This is held to be equally important if the therapist is black. Many black therapists refuse to acknowledge that the client is black in order to avoid the possible fear of weakening their own professional image and/or loss of control of the therapeutic contact.[(77)] If the black patient views himself as a second-class citizen, he is likely to consider his black therapist similarly. By introducing the subject of racial sameness at the appropriate time, the therapist can bring this important material to the forefront.

Confronting the patient in the initial interview with the racial difference between therapist and patient is not a view religiously held to by all therapists, and there is merit in allowing the issue to surface in context with the patient's own unconscious conflicts. Marked differences between patient and therapist will virtually always at some time evoke comments, whether overt or disguised. If, however, a patient questions the ability of a therapist of a different race or socioeconomic status to understand and help him, the concerns, doubts, and fears of the patient should be explored. The patient's concerns may not be primarily related to immediately apparent differences but may be an expression of his own unconscious problems or of his ambivalence to treatment and the threat of closeness. If the complaint is always taken at face value, the underlying conflict and attendant anxiety remain unknown, only to surface again in a variety of misrepresentations. Considering the fact that a therapeutic alliance can be established despite racial and other differences, it is apparent that the therapist's openness, sensitivity, and ability to empathize, together with his training and experience, are generally more important than a difference in background.[78]

The establishment of a communicative exchange is an indispensable feature of psychotherapy. The black patient who utilizes principally street talk may present a perplexing dilemma to the therapist to whom this is strange and not a part of his life experience. However, if the therapist is sincere in his interest in his patient, an inquiry will bring an explanation of what is not understood. It is not necessary for the therapist, once he gains some familiarity with the "language," to attempt to conduct interviews in street talk. Once he learns the meaning of several words or phrases he may use these as an aid in communicating, but it is crucial that the therapist be himself and not attempt to assume a role that is unnatural for him. Otherwise the patient would immediately recognize the perfidious nature of his attempt and consider his therapist to be condescending, making fun of him, or gullible—and an easy mark for manipulation.

The psychoanalytic approach seeks, in oversimplified terms, to free the patient's ego restrictions so that he has the opportunity to replace irrational responses with healthy attitudes and behavior. Central to this approach is the development and subsequent interpretation and resolution of the transference.[79] In therapy with black patients, actual transference material must be differentiated from what might be responses to the therapist's unhealthy attitudes and behavior, i.e., the countertransference phenomenon. Thomas[40] cites the two factors in classical psychoanalysis that assumedly reduce countertransference reactions: (1) The therapist's unconscious sources for psychic disturbances (blind spots) are eliminated by personal psychoanalysis; and (2) through the maintenance of an impersonal, objective aloofness, the therapist's personality does not intrude into the therapeutic situation.

The second of these two objectives, according to Frank,[80] may be both unrealistic and unattainable. He cites a variety of factors that influence the therapeutic situation, including the therapist's conviction in regard to his theory, the patient's desire to win approval from the therapist, and the ambiguity that is a result of the therapist's aloofness. These factors tend to heighten the patient's suggestibility to a number of subtle and indirect cues from the therapist—e.g., slight changes in expression, verbal intonations, movements, respiration—all of which may transmit his expectations to the patient and influence treatment without either being aware of this evasion.

In view of this delicate balance in long-term therapy, when there are racial differences, the probability of countertransference problems are markedly increased. If the therapist is unaware that the distorted responses and behavior of his patient are in response to his own attitudes, he is likely to attribute them to negative transference phenomenon. The most commonly used countertransferential mechanisms are denial, identification, overcompensation, displacement, and rationalization. They are brought into play individually as well as collectively.

Therapists who attribute all of the patient's productions as related to race as a defensive maneuver are engaging in a denial of the realities of life for black persons in America. Conversely, the therapist who accepts at face value all of what the patient says as due to racism is denying the existence of inner conflictual situations that the patient finds too anxiety-provoking to deal with.[75] This is particularly observable as resistance in therapy, when in an already established therapeutic alliance the patient switches off of the current theme and introduces new or old racial issues. Black therapists may give their patients a "rough time" for acting white while denying their own tendencies in this direction. The black therapist may react similarly toward behavior that is just the opposite in order to deny his own black identity. The black therapist might also displace his own anger toward whites onto his black patient; the patient is a less-feared target and becomes the victim of the therapist's distorted but unadmitted feelings.[77]

Another pitfall for the therapist includes his overidentification with his black patient. The white therapist may set about to prove to both his patient and himself that he is different and not a part of the racist system. Self-absorption in this effort can occur to the point of failure to confront the patient on critical issues of both an external and an internal nature. The black therapist must be exceedingly careful lest he join (or allow himself to be seduced by) his black patient in mutual commiseration over their plight. To permit this to be the sole concern is to encourage "rap sessions" with little attention paid to non-racial-associated problems. In both instances, these failures by therapists encourage acting-out behavior on the part of the patient.

The therapist who finds that, despite his oversolicitous "caring," he does not miraculously bring about expected changes in his patient may begin to question the relevancy of his training. Without seeing the "mote in his own eye," he may seek other solutions to the overwhelming problems of the disadvantaged. One apparent solution in the mid-1960s and early 1970s was to involve himself in an all-out effort at changing the social system. Thus, he actively and eagerly entered all sorts of social, political, and business efforts in the community, none of which he was equipped to handle. Such well-meaning efforts were doomed to result in failure.

SPECIAL PROBLEMS RELATED TO SOMATIC THERAPY

Thus far, treatment has been considered only from a psychotherapeutic point of view, but a comprehensive approach to patients must also include biological approaches for the relief of suffering. Research into pharmacokinetics and pharmacogenetics is in its infancy but offers promise in refining our prescribing habits. While much has yet to be learned, there is already some evidence that differences should be made in the somatic treatment of diseases unique to blacks or to which blacks are more susceptible than other ethnic groups.

Shader[46] not only lists several of these ailments but also urges psychiatrists to be more cognizant of culturally related differences when medication is used in treating minority group members. Specific reference is made to hypertension (incidence of which is high among blacks) and the need for caution in the selection of antihypertensive drugs when patients are also receiving antidepressants. In patients in sickle cell crisis, large dosages of sedative-hypnotics and the subsequent hypoxia it produces will worsen the crisis. He also indicates that sickle cell anemia patients could, if given lithium, experience difficulty since both the drug and the illness independently create problems in the reabsorption of water in the kidneys. Theoretically, the combination could have an additive affect. Experimentally, immature animals exposed to lead paint and given lithium after maturing develop irreversible central nervous system damage. This could have significant implications for poor blacks similarly exposed to lead paint in their childhood.

An array of medications of varying degrees of potency that are targeted for specific types of illness are becoming increasingly available. Not only does the prescribing physician have to accurately match drug and illness but he must be aware of the drug's effects as related to age of the patient and existent concurrent illness. He must also be knowledgeable about the antagonistic or complementary aspects of medication when other drugs are being taken, particularly in culturally related illnesses. The opportunities afforded in research in this area are not only quite evident but virtually uncontested.

SUMMATION

As in any situation where a majority group rules, the minority group has less power and fewer resources and is more greatly disadvantaged. This depicts the situation of the black minority in America. It is further apparent that the demise of slavery and the eventual changes in laws governing discrimination have not erased many culturally inculcated attitudes. Because of the long separation and isolation of the races, except for special situations dictated by whites, in-groups and out-groups are a natural development, and, as a consequence, each group develops its own stereotyped beliefs of the other. It is not then unexpected that the effects of these forces would be apparent in the mental processes and in the mental health of most persons in America. This implies that both blacks and whites alike are affected; however, this chapter is about black Americans. Perhaps a similar chapter about the psychological effects of racism on white persons in America could be written. It is probable, however, that it would be accorded little importance, since the majority of those in power are unlikely to consider any process that even suggests the possible relinquishing of their position of dominance. That this could bring about a greater good for a greater number of people is probably of little significance.

Consideration, then, of the mental health of black persons is only one facet, albeit it a significant one, of the entire complex process of racism and prejudice in America.

REFERENCES

1. A. D. Greeson, Racism and mental health, in: *Encyclopedia of Bioethics* (W. T. Reich, ed.), Free Press, Glencoe, Illinois, 1978.
2. K. B. Clark, Fifteen years of deliberate speed, in: *Annual Progress in Child Psychiatry and Child Development* (S. Chess and A. Thomas, eds.), Brunner/Mazel, New York, 1970.
3. D. P. Ausubel, Personality disorder is disease, *American Psychologist* 16:69–74, 1961.
4. T. Parsons, Definition of health and illness in the light of American values and social structure, in: *Patients, Physicians and Illness* (E. G. Jaco, ed.), Free Press, Glencoe, Illinois, 1963.
5. A. D. Schwartz, Evaluation of mental health: Three suggested approaches, *California Health* 18, 1961.
6. J. C. Baratz, *Language and cognitive assessment of Negro children: Assumptions and research needs,* Presented at the Annual Meeting of the American Psychological Association, San Francisco, 1968.
7. C. B. Wilkinson, Destructiveness of myths, *American Journal of Psychiatry* 126:1087–1092, 1970.
8. O. Petro and B. French, The black client's view of himself, *Social Casework.* October: 466–472, 1972.

9. W. A. Hayes and W. M. Banks, The nigger box or a redefinition of the counselor's role, in: *Black Psychology* (R. L. Jones, ed.), Harper & Row, New York, 1972.
10. R. Ellison, *An American Dilemma: A Review, Shadow and the Act*, Random House, New York, 1964.
11. C. Prudhomme and D. F. Musto, Historical perspective on mental health and racism in the United States, in: *Racism and Mental Health* (B. M. Kramer and B. S. Brown, eds.), University of Pittsburgh Press, Pittsburgh, 1973.
12. R. M. Stamps, *The Peculiar Institution: Slavery in the Ante-Bellum South*, Knopf, New York, 1956.
13. M. S. Cannon and B. Z. Locke, Being black is detrimental to one's mental health: Myth or reality? *Phylon* 38(4):408–428, 1977.
14. D. Wilson and E. Lantz, The effect of cultural change on the Negro race in Virginia as indicated by a study on state hospital admissions, *American Journal of Psychiatry* 114:25–32, 1957.
15. B. Pasamanick, Myths regarding prevalence of mental disease in the American Negro, *Journal of the National Medical Association* 56(1):6–17, 1964.
16. H. Pope and J. Lipinski, Diagnosis in schizophrenia and manic depressive illness, *Archives of General Psychiatry* 35:811–828, 1978.
17. R. Kleiner, J. Tuckman, and M. Lovell, Mental disorder and status based on race, *Psychiatry* 23:271–274, 1960.
18. C. Tonks, E. Paykel, and G. Klerman, Clinical depression among Negroes, *American Journal of Psychiatry* 127:329–335, 1970.
19. A. Poussaint, Black suicide, in: *Textbook of Black Related Disease* (R. Williams, ed.), McGraw-Hill, New York, 1975.
20. R. Simon, J. Fleiss, *et al.*, Depression and schizophrenia in hospitalized black and white mental patients, *Archives of General Psychiatry* 28:509–512, 1973.
21. R. I. Shader and M. Tracy, On being Black, old and emotionally troubled: How little is known, *Psychiatric Opinion* 10(6), 1973.
22. L. Bender, Behavior problems in Negro children, *Psychiatry* 2:213–228, 1939.
23. *The Negro Family: The Case for National Action*, U. S. Department of Labor, Office of Policy Planning and Research, Washington, D.C., 1965.
24. H. Biller and R. Bahm, Father absence, perceived material behavior and masculinity of self control among junior high school boys, *Developmental Psychology* 4, 1971.
25. E. M. Hetherington, Effects of paternal absence on sex type behaviors in Negro and white preadolescent males, *Journal of Personality and Social Psychology* 4, 1966.
26. M. Leichty, The absence of the father during early childhood and its effect upon the oedipal situation as reflected in young adults, *Merrill-Palmer Quarterly* 6, 1960.

27. D. Lynn and W. Sawrey, The effects of father absence on Norwegian boys and girls, *Journal of Abnormal and Social Psychology* 59, 1959.
28. T. F. Pettigrew, *A Profile of the Negro American*, Van Nostrand, Princeton, New Jersey, 1964.
29. G. Jacobson and R. Ryder, Parental loss and some characteristics of the early marriage relationship, *American Journal of Orthopsychiatry* 39, 1969.
30. L. Hunt and J. Hunt, Race and the father–son connection: The conditional relevance of father absence for the orientation and identities of adolescent boys, *Social Problems* 23, 1975.
31. C. Wilkinson, W. O'Connor, and S. Daniels, *Family studies and the treatment of black patients*, Presented at the 132nd Annual Meeting of the American Psychiatric Association, Chicago, 1979.
32. R. Rubin, Adult male absence and self-attitudes of black children, *Child Study Journal* 4:33–45, 1974.
33. E. Herzog and H. Lewis, Children in poor families, *American Journal of Orthopsychiatry* 40:375–387, 1970.
34. K. T. Mehlinger, How to retire on social security disability without really trying, *Journal of the National Medical Association* 59(1):51–54, 1967.
35. E. B. Davis and J. V. Coleman, *Interaction between community psychiatry and psychoanalysis*, Presented at the Annual Meeting of the American Psychoanalytic Association, Denver, May 3, 1974.
36. K. B. Clark, The Negro child and race prejudice, in: *Prejudice and Your Child*, Beacon, Boston, 1955.
37. M. E. Goodman, *Race Awareness in Young Children*, Collier Books, New York, 1964.
38. A. Hollingshead and F. Redlich, Social stratification and schizophrenia, *American Sociological Review* 19:302–306, 1954.
39. E. M. Goldberg and S. L. Morrison, Schizophrenia and social class, *British Journal of Psychiatry* 109:785–802, 1963.
40. A. Thomas, Pseudo-transference reactions due to cultural stereotyping, *American Journal of Orthopsychiatry* 32:894–900, 1962.
41. J. P. Comer, What happened to minorities and the poor? *Psychiatric Annals* 7(10):7996, 1977.
42. G. Alport, *The Nature of Prejudice*, Anchor Books, New York, 1958.
43. W. D. Jordan, *White over Black: American Attitudes toward the Negro*, Penguin Books, Baltimore, 1969, pp. 1550–1812.
44. C. A. Pinderhughes, Psychological and physiological origins of racism and other social discrimination, *Journal of the National Medical Association* 63(1), 1971.
45. J. Schwab, Personal communication, 1980.
46. R. I. Shader, Discussion: Cultural aspects of mental health care for black Americans: Cultural aspects of psychiatric training, in: *Cross-Cultural Psychiatry* (A. Gaw, ed.), John Wright, Littleton, Massachusetts, 1982, pp. 187–197.

47. H. Gross *et al.*, The effect of race and sex on the variation of diagnosis and disposition in a psychiatric emergency room, *Journal of Nervous and Mental Disease* 48(6):638–642, 1969.
48. A. Jackson, H. Berkowitz, and G. Farley, Race as a variable affecting the treatment involvement of children, *Journal of the American Academy of Child Psychiatry* 13(1):20–31, 1974.
49. D. Rosenthal and J. Frank, Fate of psychiatric clinic outpatients assigned to psychotherapy, *Journal of Nervous and Mental Disease* 127:330–343, 1958.
50. J. Wilder and M. Coleman, The walk-in psychiatric clinic: Some observations and follow-up, *International Journal of Social Psychiatry* 9:192–199, 1963.
51. S. Sue, D. Allen, H. McKinney, and J. Hall, *Delivery of Community Mental Health Services to Black and White Clients*, University of Washington, Seattle, 1974.
52. A. E. Raynes and G. Warren, Some distinguishing features of patients failing to attend a psychiatric clinic after referral, *American Journal of Orthopsychiatry* 41(4), 1971.
53. J. Yamamoto, Q. C. James, and N. Pailey, Cultural problems in psychiatric therapy, *Archives of General Psychiatry* 19:4549, 1969.
54. B. G. Fiman, *Special Report on Inequities in Mental Health Service Delivery*, Prepared for the National Institute of Mental Health Center for Study of Minority Group Mental Health Programs, Human Sciences Research, Inc., March 1975.
55. R. Warren *et al.*, Differential attitudes of black and white patients toward psychiatric treatment in a child guidance clinic, *American Journal of Orthopsychiatry* 42(2):301–302, 1972.
56. R. W. Reddick, *Addition Rates to Federally Funded Community Mental Health Centers, United States, 1973*, Mental Health Statistical Note No. 126, U. S. Department of Health, Education and Welfare, Public Health Service, Alcohol, Drug Abuse and Mental Health Administration, National Institute of Mental Health, Division of Biometry and Epidemiology, Survey and Reports Branch.
57. L. K. Brown, Psychotherapy: Black and white, *Journal of the National Medical Association* 64(1):19–22, 1972.
58. J. B. Deregowski, Effect of cultural value of time and recall, *British Journal of Social and Clinical Psychology* 9:37–41, 1970.
59. F. C. Bartlett, *Remembering: A Study in Experimental and Social Psychology*, Cambridge University Press, Cambridge, Massachusetts, 1932, pp. 253.
60. C. B. Wilkinson, Growing up in the ghetto, in: *Current Issues in Adolescent Psychiatry* (J. C. Schoolar, ed.), Brunner/Mazel, New York, 1973.
61. C. J. Sager, T. L. Brayboy, and B. R. Waxenberg, Black patient–white therapist, *American Journal of Orthopsychiatry* 42(3):415–423, 1972.
62. S. Chess, K. B. Clark, and A. Thomas, Importance of cultural evaluation in psychiatric diagnosis and treatment, *Psychiatric Quarterly* 27(102), 1953.

63. W. Bradshaw, Personal communication, July 1979.
64. W. Grier and P. Cobbs, *Black Rage*, Basic Books, New York, 1968.
65. C. Reed, Personal communication, 1977.
66. S. Parker and R. J. Kleiner, *Mental Illness in the Urban Negro Community*, Free Press, New York, 1966.
67. P. M. Blau, Social mobility and interpersonal relations, *American Sociology Review* 21:290, 1956.
68. L. W. Warner, The society, the individual and his mental disorders, *American Journal of Psychiatry* 94:274, 1937.
69. S. M. Lipset and R. Bendix, *Social Mobility in Industrial Society*, University of California Press, Berkeley of Los Angeles, 1963, pp. 64–72, 251–252.
70. R. J. Kleiner and O. G. Dalgard, Social mobility and psychiatric disorders: A reevaluation and interpretation, *American Journal of Psychotherapy* 29:150–165, 1975.
71. J. Ruesch, *Chronic Disease and Psychological Invalidism: A Psychosomatic Study, American Society for Research in Psychosomatic Problems*, New York, 1946, pp. 104–124.
72. T. H. Holmes, Life situations, emotions and disease, *Psychosomatics* 19(12):747–754, 1978.
73. E. Durkheim, *Suicide*, Free Press, Glencoe, Illinois, 1957.
74. R. Waite, The Negro patient and clinical theory, *Journal of Consulting and Clinical Psychology* 32:427–433, 1968.
75. W. H. Bradshaw, Training psychiatrists for working with blacks in basic residency program, *American Journal of Psychiatry* 135:1520–1524.
76. J. H. Carter, Frequent mistakes made with black patients in psychotherapy, *Journal of the National Medical Association* 71:1007–1009, 1979.
77. M. Calnek, Racial factors in the countertransference: The black therapist and the black client, *American Journal of Orthopsychiatry* 40:39–46, 1970.
78. C. A. Pinderhughes and E. B. Pinderhughes, Prospective of training directors, in: *Cross-Cultural Psychiatry* (A. Gaw, ed.), John Wright-PSG Inc., Boston, 1982.
79. E. Chance, Transference in group therapy, *International Journal of Group Psychotherapy* 1:40, 1952.
80. J. D. Frank, The psychodynamics of the psychotherapeutic relationship, *Psychiatry* 22:17, 1959.

3

Hispanics

PSYCHIATRIC ISSUES

CERVANDO MARTINEZ, JR.

INTRODUCTION

The Hispanic people in the United States are a large, diverse, and increasingly important political group. The name Hispanic is used because most are of Spanish descent and also because, to varying degrees, the Spanish language is central to their identity. This group includes New York and island Puerto Ricans, Cuban Americans, Mexican Americans, and others. The "others" are the smallest group, which includes people from Central and South American countries, the Caribbean, and Spain. The term *Latino* has also been used to describe the Hispanic minority; *Chicano* is a term of pride and self-identification used by some Mexican Americans. According to the 1980 census there are 14.6 million Spanish-speaking or Hispanic Americans in the continental United States and over 3 million island Puerto Ricans. The largest subgroups

CERVANDO MARTINEZ, JR. • Department of Psychiatry, The University of Texas Health Science Center at San Antonio, San Antonio, Texas 78284.

are the Mexican Americans, the Puerto Ricans, and the Cuban Americans, in that order. Mexican Americans are estimated to represent upwards of 60% of *hispanos*. Because of higher birth rates and continued immigration some projections have Hispanics surpassing blacks numerically by 1990.

In this discussion, Hispanic will refer primarily to Mexican Americans, Puerto Ricans, and Cubans. The mental health literature related to Hispanics is growing rapidly[1,2] and mostly covers these three groups, especially Mexican Americans. The literature has evolved and its growth began to be particularly evident in the 1970s. During the 1940s and 1950s research studies in the literature were mostly psychological or anthropological. The psychological studies were usually comparative studies of intelligence testing involving Hispanic adults and children, and usually concluded that Hispanics (Mexican Americans were the group usually tested) were of inferior intelligence because their intelligence test scores were lower than those of Anglos. The effect of bilingualism on IQ testing and the fact that the people tested spoke English as a second language did not deter these investigators from their stigmatizing conclusions. Some early anthropological studies also presented findings that tended to stereotype Hispanics as fatalistic, lazy, and content. The literature of the 1960s, especially that involving Mexican Americans, was partly a response to these earlier works and served to undo some of the stereotypes that had become behavioral science lore. Some of these works of the 1960s also served to outline important issues that needed further study, such as the problem of underutilization of mental health services by Hispanics. During the 1970s there appeared a fairly impressive body of literature on psychopathology, language, therapy, and service delivery. These works, however, are still only a beginning. There is a need for additional well-done cross-cultural, epidemiological studies, further exploration of ethnic differences in response to different therapeutic modalities, and comparative physiologic studies.

Although these three Hispanic groups have many things in common, they should be distinguished from one another. First, they differ in the reasons and circumstances of being here. Puerto Ricans are all U.S. citizens, and many have come to the mainland seeking a better life and now constitute a significant portion of several northeastern cities (e.g., New York, Boston). This migration continues in both directions and has enabled them to maintain their culture and language. For most Puerto Ricans, life in the United States has also been a life of poverty. Finally, Puerto Ricans vary from those that look "white," and are of more direct Spanish descent, to black Puerto Ricans.

Most Cuban Americans came to the United States during and after the Cuban revolution and more recently during the relaxation of the prohibition on immigration. Many have prospered in the South Florida area, and although there has been some assimilation, they successfully maintain their language and cultural heritage.

Mexican Americans are both immigrants and descendants of the original settlers of the Southwest. Groups in New Mexico and Colorado are direct descendants of the Spanish colonists. The majority, however, are of Mexican descent; that is, they are a *mestizo* people, the product of the blending of the Spanish and the Indian, physically and culturally. In addition, the Mexican Americans in the Southwest, like the blacks, have been the victims of official discrimination and segregation in schools, jobs, the ballot box, and public places. Because of Mexico's own underdevelopment and the above repressive forces, Mexican Americans have also been a largely poor group.

The most important thing that Hispanics have in common is the use and influence of the Spanish language. As would be expected, there is great variation in the extent of Spanish language use among *hispanos;* however, the majority are bilingual to varying degrees, and contrary to the expectations of advocates of the melting pot, the use of Spanish will most likely continue. Spanish use has been and will be strong because of continued migration and renewed ethnic pride. The use of formal and informal tenses in Spanish also affects behavior and will be discussed below.

Finally, *hispanos* share a common cultural heritage, again with intergroup differences. They are predominantly Catholic, they are family- and extended-family-centered, and they adhere to Latin customs and codes in interpersonal relations. Some of the cultural factors effect health and mental health behavior.

CULTURAL CONSIDERATIONS

The culture of Hispanic Americans includes not only important elements of Spanish culture but also Indian and African influences. Puerto Rican and Cuban American culture is a blend of Spanish and Afro-Caribbean features; Mexican American culture is a mixture of Spanish and Mexican Indian influences. It goes without saying that all three groups are strongly affected by the dominant and powerful American culture. Within each of the three groups there are subgroups that vary in the extent of acculturation, depending on generation of birth, place of upbringing, immigration patterns, parental habits, socioeconomic status, and personal choice. Variation in extent of acculturation is reflected in the use of the Spanish language. That is, the more assimilated the person is into "American" culture, the more likely he is to lose the use of Spanish. However, this generalization is not so simple for two reasons: Spanish is one of the more tenacious languages in the world, and Hispanics, unlike European ethnic groups, are being continuously replenished by Spanish-speaking immigrants from Puerto Rico, Mexico, and, more recently, Cuba. Since a great deal of what is "cultural" is tied up in the language (some have even said that culture *is* language), it is important to state a few generalizations about the Spanish language as a prelude to other considerations. Like other ethnic groups in the United States today, Hispanics are making conscious attempts to maintain their cultural and linguistic identity and individuality.

The influence of the Spanish language has general and specific effects. The language has formal and informal tenses for objects and verbs—e.g., *usted* ("you"—formal) and *tu* ("you"—informal, intimate) both mean you. The *tu* form is used when referring to younger people and close acquaintances. These characteristics of the language plus other factors lead to a certain formalism in interpersonal relations. This is not to say that all Hispanics rigidly adhere to the above usages in daily discourse; they don't. This quality of the language adds an emphasis to style, manners, and propriety in interpersonal relations. Thus, with the Hispanic patient, the clinician should be somewhat more formal and avoid too rapid a progression to a first-name informal relationship.

There is a paradox here, though, because there is also importance placed on *personalismo*,—that is, concern about personal attention, personal contacts, and similar factors. Some have even indicated that the term *la platica* ("the chat") be used to describe the interview with the Hispanic. The paradox, however, is not so complete. Hispanics do appreciate informality, personal interest, and chatting, but only after the proper formal amenities have been considered and respected.

Two other important cultural characteristics are the great emphasis placed on close family ties and the stricter definition of roles, especially sexual ones. A great deal has been said and written about the importance of the family in Hispanic interpersonal relations.[3]. This is a key consideration in clinical work with Hispanics: when attempting hospitalization, when trying to mobilize social support, and when understanding family psychodynamics. Like many other ethnic groups (e.g., Italians), Hispanics place great value on maintaining close family ties. Godparents (*compadres*) are still widely promoted and include *compadres* through marriage (attendants) and *compadres* through baptism of children. One important example of how awareness of this important cultural characteristic can help in clinical practice should be mentioned: working with the poorly motivated patient. Locating a godparent *compadre* or *comadre* and soliciting his or her support in encouraging treatment can often mean the difference in getting a resistive patient to accept needed care.

Despite the rapid and powerful changes occurring in the definition of sexual and family roles in American society, many Hispanic families remain very traditional in their views of these matters. This traditional view of family roles has been described repeatedly among all Hispanic groups studied. In the more traditional Hispanic family the father's role is strictly defined as that of main provider, protector, and breadwinner. The wife's role involves care of the children and the home. Working outside the home is discouraged. These values are reinforced by the predominant Catholic beliefs of most Hispanic families, by their greater number of children per family, and by the social and economic realities of a life in poverty. Adherence to "traditional" roles does not mean belief in *machismo,* a term used to describe the male belief in his superiority. There is no evidence that Hispanic males are more inclined to infidelity or wife beating than non-Hispanics. The more traditional family role definition does set the stage for family conflicts resulting from changing, modern role expectations. Intrafamily conflicts about values and behavior tend to be more keen and intense.

> Paula, a 22-year-old woman recovering from a prolonged schizophrenic disorder, experienced added difficulty during the intermediate phase of her treatment because of intense conflict and resulting arguments with her parents. This conflict occurred because, among other things, there were very wide differences of opinion about appropriate dating behavior and traveling alone. Although fairly young, the parents, both born in Mexico, still held very traditional views about the behavior of young adults. Paula's views, conservative by some standards, were too extreme for them. The therapist in this case had to consider that although the parents' views seemed outdated and rigid, they were not out of keeping with the views of other Hispanics and had to be taken into account.

The tighter family relations and the tendency for family members to rely on one another for various types of assistance (the extended family) have effects, good and bad, on the mental health of individual members. The close family can be a source of support for the stressed or decompensating individual. It has been speculated that this supportive-therapeutic effect of the close Hispanic family is one reason why Hispanics tend to be underrepresented in mental health clinics. On the other hand, the emphasis on close family ties, like the stricter definition of family roles, can have pathological interpersonal effects, such as the breeding of excessive dependency.

These cultural characteristics are not the only ones that have mental health implications. They are mentioned to illustrate two points: that Hispanic Americans carry a different culture baggage than Americans of nothern European ancestry, and that many of these peculiarly Hispanic cultural characteristics have implications for clinical practice. Students of ethnic groups in America can correctly argue that many of these characteristics (e.g., close families) are shared by other immigrant groups, especially southern European ones. What will probably continue to distinguish Hispanics from these other ethnic groups will be the preservation of their language by a process of cultural diffusion from Latin American to North American. The processes of acculturation and assimilation will be balanced by replenishment and renewal through immigration.

CLINICAL DIAGNOSIS AND PSYCHOPATHOLOGY

There is general agreement that most psychiatric disorders have roughly the same incidence and prevalance throughout the world. Until recently it was thought that bipolar disorder and schizophrenia differed in incidence and prevalence on the two sides of the Atlantic. It has now been demonstrated that these differences were due to different diagnostic criteria used by clinicians in the United States and Europe. Disorders due to malnutrition and other somatic causes may occur at different rates in different countries as a result of the level of economic development and other factors. Thus, for Hispanics in the United States it would be expected that they would suffer from the major functional disorders at approximately the same rate as other Americans. There is little evidence to contradict this view. Over 20 years ago Jaco [4] studied the rate of psychiatric hospitilization for psychosis (including the organic ones) for Mexican Americans in Texas and found a lower rates than for Anglos and blacks. Rate of hospitalization, however, is not a good indicator of incidence, particularly for this ethnic group living close to the Mexican border (where to this day many go for medical care) and in a state that practiced official discrimination in public places until the 1960s. Other studies,[5,6] however, have demonstrated underutilization of psychiatric services (both inpatient and outpatient) by Hispanics. Underutilization of services also does not necessarily mean lower incidence and prevalence, but more likely reflects institutional barriers (language, racism), better family supports, use of other resources (folk healers, priests), data-gathering methods, or shunting into the penal systems. These many epidemiologic questions continue to remain unanswered.

There is no doubt, however, that the form the functional psychoses and other disorders take among Hispanics is different from that among other Americans. It has been fairly well demonstrated that sociocultural elements weave themselves into patients' delusions—for example, religious and scientific themes. Among Hispanics, elements of the Catholic faith and folk medical beliefs often are incorporated into the content of thinking of disturbed individuals. In addition, there is evidence that there may be specific "cultural bound" syndromes among Hispanics (see Puerto Rican syndrome below).

Among the organic disorders and the sociopsychobiological conditions (alcoholism and drug addiction) the situation is more complicated, and there are few data to help. It can be postulated that Hispanics, being overrepresented among the poor in the United States, are recipients of a lower level of health care, especially prenatal maternal care and infant care, than the average American and thus would suffer from a higher incidence of birth complications. This is the case in studies done along the Mexican border, where, in counties with large Mexican American populations, the infant mortality rate is higher than in counties farther from the border. The counties near the boarder are also poorer. Mexico, a developing country but still a poor one, reports a higher incidence of epilepsy than the United States, presumably because of its poorer economic status and less-developed health care resources. Comparative rates for epilepsy, organic brain damage, and severe mental retardation in Hispanic children have not been reported, to my knowledge.

Comparative rates for heroin addiction between Mexican Americans and other groups have been reported[7,8] and indicate that there is a much higher than expected rate among Hispanics. The reasons for this marked difference are not known but probably involve issues of drug availability, poverty, law enforcement, and perhaps tradition. (There is a long tradition of the use of psychotropic substances in some Mexican Indian groups.) Studies on the relative prevalence of alcoholism among Hispanics, although open to criticism on methodological grounds, also indicate a great prevalence of this complex disorder among Hispanics.[9] Finally, toxic inhalant abuse (spray paints, aerosols), especially among Mexican American children, is a serious (and until recently an almost completely ignored) mental health, school, and community problem. It is estimated that Chicano children are 14 times more likely to abuse toxic inhalants than their non-Hispanic peers.

Regardless of what social psychiatric studies suggest about the occurrence of the various disorders among Hispanics, the clinician is still ultimately faced with the tasks of evaluating the single individual, in his social and cultural environment, and responding therapeutically. In the process of this work the clinician is presented with two basic intervening variables: language and culture. It should be self-evident that if an individual who primarily speaks one language undergoes a diagnostic psychiatric interview in another, there may occur distorting effects caused by this language discrepancy. The interweaving of cultural factors into this process further complicates matters.

However, the situation is not quite so simple. The degree of bilingualism in any group varies a great deal; at the extremes are those individuals who speak only one language with any degree of fluency. The majority, however, are "bilingual" or have some significant degree of fluency in both languages, but may perfer one to the other. There are also many truly bilingual persons. The work of Marcos and some of the comments that follow refer to those Hispanics who perfer Spanish or speak only minimal or no English. In these individuals, the clinician should pay particularly close attention to the effect of language on the diagnostic process. When a person thinks in one language and then speaks in another there occur certain changes that can be interpreted as psychopathological. There is hesitation and groping for words that can appear as blocking, thought derailment, or lossening of associations. A limited vocabulary in a new language results in a simpler, restricted verbal output. This may be seen as impoverishment of thought or concreteness. The expression of complex thought is blunted. This can effect judgments about intelligence and cognition.

Language spoken can also have significant effects on the description, expression, and manifestation of emotions. It is difficult enough, even when both the patient and the therapist speak the same language, to assess and understand emotions. Simply identifying and labeling an emotional response may prove difficult across a language gulf. The expression of an emotion may likewise be affected by the process of translation and expression into another language. To have to undergo psychiatric evaluation and treatment in a language other than one's own is probably distressing to most individuals. This situational anxiety adds a further complicating factor. It may effect the expression of thought and emotion, and it may bring out certain behavioral or "state" changes that can also lead to mislabeling.

In women, hysterical traits may become evident. These may consist of coyness, negativism, and apparent excessive use of denial. These changes in behavior, in an individual struggling with a new language, may not necessarily be indicative of a personality disorder but may be a conseqence of the anxiety produced by the language difference. In men, one may see negativism, hostility, or excessive passivity. In addition, it has been noted that Mexican males wear a mask to hide their true feelings and to reduce their vulnerability. This may also influence the evaluation of affective response.

The use of an interpreter in the diagnostic situation remains controversial. For several reasons the traditional wisdom has advised against the use of the interpreter except when absolutely necessary. The interpreter brings a third person into the process. This has usually been seen as producing negative effects because of a supposed greater likelihood for distortion and misinterpretation. Also, patients are reported to find it disagreeable. A recent report,[(10)] however, questions whether the use of the interpreter invariably has negative effects. The patients studied by these workers saw the use of the interpreter positively, as evidence of interest and concern for better communication and understanding. It seems reasonable to conclude that, like any other tool used in diagnosis, the interpreter may have variable effects and these need to be taken into account in the interpretation of clinical findings.

The work of Marcos *et al.*[(11)] has been helpful in clarifying the effects of language of interview on the findings on the mental status exam. Marcos has shown that, when patients whose primary language is Spanish but who are bilingual (they speak English also) are interviewed in English, they demonstrate findings in thinking processes and affect indicative of psychopathology. Specifically, when interviewed in English these patients demonstrate loosening of associations, blocking, and other clinical signs usually interpreted as abnormal. In English their affective range seems restricted and blunted. When interviewed in Spanish these same patients demonstrate markedly fewer abnormalities in both areas, thinking and affect. The study was done on schizophrenics and did not imply that when they were interviewed in Spanish the psychopathology disappeared. It did not; it only diminished.

Some workers[12,13] have reported that Hispanic patients differ from non-Hispanics in the type of presenting symptomatology they demonstrate. Specifically mentioned are somatic symptoms such as headaches and pain in the back of the neck (*la nuca*). This observation is consistent with that of other clinicians; however, it is not clear whether this is a typically Hispanic characteristic or is more related to socioeconomic level. In large-scale mental health surveys (e.g., the Midtown Manhattan Study) it has been found that people from lower economic groups have a greater tendency to manifest anxiety via somatic symptoms. The poor are also more likely to experience stress due to overcrowding, lack of material necessities, and financial uncertainty. Hispanics, like blacks, are overrepresented among the poor.

Syndromes specific to Hispanics have also been described. The most common one is the Puerto Rican syndrome[14] or *Ataque.*[15] This is a syndrome of a hysterical nature, characterized by sudden seizurelike activity and thought to serve to defend against overwhelming aggressive impulses. Various clinicians have stated that this type of conversion symptom pattern is more common among Puerto Ricans, but no quantitative studies to support this clinical impression have been done.

Thus, in the diagnostic assessment of a Hispanic patient, the clinician has to take into account language and cultural factors. This does not mean, as some have maintained, that a Hispanic cannot be correctly diagnosed by a non-Hispanic. What does obtain is that the diagnostic process is more complex when additional language and cultural factors have to be taken into account. One cultural component frequently present that may compound diagnostic thinking is the belief in folk illnesses and therapies.

These culturally specific beliefs will not be fully reviewed here because good descriptions in detail have been published elsewhere.[16,17] However, they do have specific and important psychiatric implications that deserve special attention. Almost all cultural, ethnic, or racial groups have folk health beliefs and practices which are adhered to despite acculturation/assimilation, and which operate in parallel to beliefs and practices in scientific medical systems. In some countries (e.g., China) the scientific medical system has learned from and used elements of the traditional (folk) system. Many Hispanics likewise continue to believe in and practice certain folk medical traditions.

The continued presence of these beliefs manifests itself in clinical psychiatric practice in several ways. Probably the least common way is when the folk belief is part of a delusional system. This must be distinguished, of course, from the simple yet strongly held belief, not of a delusional nature, in the phenomenon at hand. Some Hispanics believe in hexes, spirits, and voodoo. These are not delusions; rather they are culturally sanctioned beliefs. The determination as to whether a particular belief is part of a delusional system has to include an assessment of other factors in the history and the findings on mental status consistent with psychosis.

The most common clinical manifestation of these beliefs is their presence as part of the patient's or family's struggle to explain and cope with the presence of a serious and often baffling psychiatric disorder. There is a human tendency to seek an explanation for severe and difficult-to-comprehend illnesses such as cancer, epilepsy, and psychosis, and for these aliments, resort to faith healers is well known. Similarly, Hispanics often seek an explanation for psychiatric disorders from the *espiritista* (Puerto Rican) or *curandera* (Mexican American). These are folk healers who use a variety of techniques (religious, ritualistic, herbal, manipulative) and who are used extensively by Hispanics who have faith in their ministrations, or who during a period of personal confusion seek a more understandable or less threatening explanation for their problems.

> A young Mexican American man had been acting bizarrely for several months prior to evaluation in a rural health clinic. His family had first taken him to be treated by a *curandera* (folk healer) because they believed that his change in behavior was due to a hex (*mal puesto*) placed on him by a rejected girlfriend who was jealous and hurt. There was transient improvement after the first visit to the *curandera*; however, subsequent consultations were of less benefit, and he was eventually brought to the health clinic, where he was considered to be experiencing an acute schizophrenic psychosis.

This vignette illustrates several points. First of all, it underlines the well-known observation that the families of patients undergoing puzzling health changes will search and use whatever resources are closest at hand. In this case, in a rural area near the Mexican border, a *curandera* was consulted first, but when her treatment proved ineffective, help was sought through the medical care system. The initial improvement reported may have been a placebolike effect generated as a result of the patient's and family's strong faith in the healer. Some folk healers are quite dramatic, others very supportive—both of which may take advantage of specific psychological needs in their clients. The mention of jealousy as a motive for a hex being placed is also characteristic of rural Mexicans and may be explained on the basis of the Hispanic tendency to suppress or project an expression of anger. It has also been noted that Hispanics may utilize both the folk and scientific medical systems concurrently for the same disorder or for different problems. Folk healers are commonly consulted for treatment of chronic painful, mildly disabling conditions such as musculoskeletal disorders, anxiety states with physiologic manifestations, and cholelithiasis.

THERAPY

There exists a major dilemma in the area of therapy with Hispanics: This is a large group in America that still speaks mainly Spanish, yet there are few Spanish-speaking mental health professionals to provide services. In the schools this dilemma posed by the language has been partially dealt with by means of bilingual programs. (Bilingual public school programs involve the teaching of school material in the child's "other" language in order to lessen the difficulty of having to learn new school material and English simultaneously. These programs are controversial. Proponents see them as aiding children to remain in school and learn better. Opponents feel that they promote separation and retard learning of English.) No such large-scale effort has been attempted in the area of mental health services—an area where proper communication is paramount. Although there have been efforts by the federal government and some graduate schools to increase the number of Hispanic mental health professionals, the number is still low,[18] or as in the case of psychiatrists, those that exist are poorly distributed. The problems encountered in making a proper diagnosis when working with a bilingual patient have already been described, and the situation is even more serious in the area of psychiatric treatment where there are two basic modalities: talk and drugs. It should be self-evident that the efficacy of a verbal therapy, whether it is counseling, analytically oriented psychotherapy, or group psychotherapy, is compromised if adequate communication does not take place. If communication is poor, even pharmacotherapy is liable to be less effective through diminution of the placebo effect or poor compliance due to faulty explanation of proper drug use.

Two additional problems complicate the situation further: economic status and cultural understanding. Hispanics not only speak another language but also tend to be poor. The myth in psychiatric circles that poor people are poor candidates for psychotherapy has been pretty well debunked,[19] but it still affects the planning and selection of patients by many programs and clinicians. Thus, Hispanics are working under a double burden when seeking mental health care; others would say it is a triple burden—i.e., cultural factors.

In reality, the picture is not so bleak as it is complicated by the above factors. Some Hispanics are adequately fluent in English and many are quite acculturated and middle class in orientation. This more English-fluent, acculturated group of Hispanics, although presenting fewer of the problems described above, nevertheless should not be viewed as totally like Anglo-Americans. There are several issues worth keeping in mind when working with the more acculturated, English-speaking Hispanics.

The first is that these Hispanic's greater degree of acculturation and assimilation can itself produce conflicts of several types and lead to specific problems. The more acculturated individual may develop serious identity conflicts, anxiety, and other symptomatic behavior as a result of a too rapid shedding of the traditional Hispanic cultural values, beliefs, and habits. Some of these traditional attitudes include the belief in the father and males as dominant in the family, and the expectation that children remain close to home. Also included are a host of cultural traditions ranging from those dealing with the use of the language to others having to do with eating. Particularly now that there is a heightened consciousness about ethnic identity among Hispanics, those that have acculturated in too rapid and perhaps too extreme a fashion may feel acutely conflicted and make desperate efforts to reembrace their culture or flee and deny it. Both extremes can be problematic.

Rapid acculturation also leaves the individual susceptible to serious conflict with parents and other less acculturated relatives, with resulting interpersonal friction, alienation from a valuable support system, and other difficulties. It has been demonstrated in other ethnic groups that the second generation of immigrants has a higher suicide rate than the first. One of the postulated reasons for this is the culture conflict and alienation described above. Thus, when working with the more acculturated Hispanic, the therapist should not assume that ethnicity and cultural identification are no longer issues; they obviously can very much be issues of central concern and should be explored. Often what is experienced by the Hispanic patient is a great deal of remorse and longing for the lost language and culture. Frustration and shame are common, especially in the presence of more traditional Spanish-speaking peers, and sometimes there is a great deal of anger, resentment, and misunderstanding of parents who did not teach their children Spanish in the home. The parents may have sincerely believed that they were doing the best for their children by helping them to become fluent in English without the supposed interference of Spanish, only to find that now Spanish is valued, and as a result they are held to blame for their way of upbringing. Often, second-generation Hispanics, particularly Mexican Americans, are not fully aware of the racism and other pressures on their parents during the 1930s, 1940s and 1950s that made them try to deny their language and heritage.

Understanding aspects of the culture, even when working with acculturated Hispanics, is therefore useful. It is especially important that the therapist remember the strong traditional beliefs still prevalent among Hispanics, especially those beliefs having to do with strict definition of family roles, sex roles, and health. In practice this means that the therapist must be aware that suggestions for change, especially in the woman, in the direction of greater personal freedom and autonomy may be met by strong resistance and conflict. The spouse and other family members may also be opposed to such movement. It is a common error of therapists working with Hispanic women to encourage too eagerly a sense of independence in a woman and family who are still deeply caught up in traditional beliefs about the roles of men and women.

There are several perspectives or approaches that can be used when working with persons from a different cultural group. One approach is the one already mentioned, which involved assessing the acculturation level of the individual—say, along a traditional-modern continuum—and attempting to understand conflict in terms of internal or interpersonal value conflict. Of course, one assumes that in all individuals there are conflict areas that are universal but not necessarily free of cultural influence, such as conflicts about dependence and independence. These "human" conflicts can be intensified, diminished, modulated, and shaped by cultural factors. For example, the conflict in adolescents involving dependence and independence may be intensified in the Hispanic female if the family still adheres to the more rigid traditional beliefs about the behavior of women.

Another perspective that may be useful is the "explanatory model" approach.[(20)] Using this approach, the therapist explores and understands the patient's "explanation" for his or her condition. Therapy then departs from and utilizes the patient's explanatory model. Psychotherapy involving therapist and patient from roughly the same sociocultural group usually proceeds on the basis of certain shared assumptions:

that previous historical events influence present behavior, that talking helps, that emotional conflict may produce physical symptoms, that certain emotional problems are health problems. In working across cultural boundaries, there may be fewer or different shared assumption; e.g., Hispanics commonly believe that certain symptoms (anxiety, insomnia) are due to hexes (withcraft) or bad spirits. In other cases, symptoms may be attributed to an episode of uncontrolled anger or a demonstration of disrespect for elders. Therapeutic wisdom says that therapist–patient expectations should be properly aligned and congruent for therapy to work. When one is working across cultures, this alignment of perspectives may not always be possible. The therapist may have to be satisfied with simply understanding the patient's explanatory model of dysfunction, or the therapist may need to utilize the patient's explanatory language to more effectively produce change.

Likewise, many Hispanics may simultaneously use two modes of thinking (explaining): the folk and the scientific. Many Puerto Ricans continue using *espiritistas*. These are individuals who are supposed to have healing powers and who follow the principles of *espiritismo*, a complex belief system that attributes various states of ill health (physical and mental) and interpersonal problems to the intervention of different kinds of *espiritos* (spirits). Relief is sought from *espiritistas* who have seancelike group functions where some of the mechanisms of group therapy come into play. The therapist working with Puerto Rican patients should not only be aware of the existence of this belief system but should also, if necessary, be prepared to function within both systems. The following clinical vignette from Comas-Diaz[21] exemplifies this point.

> Mr. E. is a 39-year-old married man living with his wife and children. He used to work as an unskilled factory worker. He stopped working 7 years ago because he

could not perform his working duties. He was diagnosed as emotionally disturbed and was being supported by Social Security disability insurance. The client had deteriorated to the point that he was no longer able to perform social roles. He was referred for treatment with a diagnosis of schizophrenia, paranoid type. During the initial interview, the client was accompanied by his wife, who acted as informant. She stated that he was suffering from "hearing and seeing things" and severe insomnia, and that he needed medication in order to sleep. After a psychiatric evaluation, the client was prescribed an antipsychotic and a hypnotic, and was referred for ongoing psychotherapy. During the course of treatment, the client revealed that he was seeing *celajes,* which were *animas* (souls) of people that he had killed in self-defense. The client was very afraid of those *espiritos intranquilos* because he believed that they were after him. Individual therapy was focused on the client's feelings of guilt. In addition, couple therapy was provided to work on the client's marital conflicts. The therapist provided a structure in which the client could safely ventilate his fears and work out his guilt. She (the therapist) also supported his strong belief in *espiritismo* and, for example, reinforced his decision to wear a *resguardo* to obtain spiritual protection. The therapist did not question the client's world view and supported his attempts at paying his debt to the intranquil spirits by helping them fulfill their spiritual mission through burning candles, saying prayers, etc., as a means of dealing with anxiety. In this way, the issues of responsibility and guilt were worked within the two belief systems in order to assist the client to regain some control over his life.

This case history, like the one presented in an earlier section, illustrates how the Hispanic patient's cultural beliefs may interweave themselves into the processes of diagnosis and treatment. The examiner should first be aware that these beliefs exist and that they commonly manifest themselves in psychiatric (as well as general health) settings; however, what is or is not done after recognizing that the beliefs are held depends on the clinical situation. There are cases where holding the folk belief is used as a form of pathological denial, and it may be indicated that the therapist try to counter the belief or discourage the use of the folk systems. Often, however, the Hispanic patient and family can use both systems without apparent discomfort.

The conduct of psychotherapy with Hispanic patients poses obvious problems if the patient speaks no English or if English is a poor second language. Many Hispanics born in the United States speak Spanish at home as a first language; later they learn English, but their English remains rather rudimentary. It goes without saying that psychotherapy in these situations can be more difficult, but also more challenging. The two individuals involved in the psychotherapeutic endeavor have to understand each other clearly if the effort is to have a chance to succeed. One has to remember that many Hispanics are thinking in Spanish, translating to themselves, then verbalizing in English. Much can be lost in translation. However, the extra care and attention paid to clarification may (and should) come across as added empathy and thus enhance the therapeutic task.

The use of interpreters in psychotherapy with Hispanic patients who speak absolutely no English is difficult to assess. The paper by Kline *et al.*,[10] cited earlier, analyzed patients' responses to the use of an interpreter and found that patients didn't necessarily respond negatively. The authors speculated that their patients' positive response to therapeutic interactions involving interpreters may have been because the patients saw the careful use of interpreters as a sign of concern and interest by the therapist. From this it could be concluded that some of the nonverbal aspects of the therapeutic interaction came through and indeed might be enhanced with the use of interpreters. There could be merit in using bilingual workers (therapists?) as interpreters and cotherapists in group therapy. Examples of this from our experience in several therapeutic groups appear worth mentioning. The first of these is the use of Spanish in simultaneous or parallel translation by the Spanish-speaking staff and/or patients. We have noted that if English is the language being used by the majority of patients and there is no translating going on, those patients who speak little or no English may still benefit from the groups. They may be able to understand a significant amount, speak some, and obtain benefit even if the entire process is in English. When Spanish is permitted for clarification or amplification, this tends to further improve communication. When bilingual therapists are available and patient demand justifies their use, groups only in Spanish can be formed. This, however, presents problems of a different sort—e.g., therapists have to be flexible in their own use of Spanish, recognizing, as in English, that there are many types of Spanish and that the bilingual therapist has to respect the idioms of all Hispanics. The therapists also have to be sensitive about the feelings of very acculturated Hispanics who may join a Spanish-speaking group only to find that they have difficulty understanding or communicating because of their own limitations.

At a minimum, the therapist intending to work with Spanish-speaking patients should master the pronunciation of Spanish names. Correct pronunciation of a patient's name conveys interest and concern. Some Hispanic patients, due to anxiety, fear, shame, or anger, may present themselves as able to speak less English than is actually the case. The sensitive interviewer shouldn't let the patient's demurral lead to the conclusion that further communication is not possible.

Sensitively provided reassurance, exploration of the underlying emotions, or clarification of some confusion may cause the reluctant Hispanic patient to drop this defensive use of ignorance of English.

Once the Hispanic patient is engaged in psychotherapy, most of the issues to be explored will be no different from those found in all human beings. Some more problematic areas related to cultural factors have been mentioned previously (intensified conflict about roles and family ties). There are some suggestions in the literature that specific types of psychotherapy may be more efficacious with Hispanics. The more directive approaches have appeared to work well. It is unclear, however, whether this is a selective effect, since comparative studies of various types of psychotherapy have not been done.

One specific treatment modality should be mentioned: the Spanish-speaking intermediate care program. In many communities with significant Hispanic populations, it may be feasible and therapeutically indicated to establish some form of intermediate care program for Hispanic patients recovering from severe psychiatric disorders. Most institutions would probably not have the demand or resources for a full-fledged Hispanic inpatient unit; nor is it clinically practical to concentrate Spanish-speaking personnel solely at the point in the therapeutic process where the patient is most disturbed, least in contact with reality, and least amenable to verbal intervention. It is far more productive to establish Spanish-speaking programs that can intervene at a later point, when the patient is more in contact. A program can be a complete inpatient installation, as is the Chicano Unit of 90 beds at the San Antonio State Hospital; it can be a day program within an institution, similar to that at St. Elizabeth's Hospital, Washington, D.C.; or it might be simply a group for Spanish-speaking recovering psychotics. The objective is to intervene in a timely manner, in the appropriate language, during the course of a psychotic illness to prevent gross "sealing over," promote self-awareness and insight into illness, and strengthen ego resources.

It is particularly important when working with severly ill Hispanic patients to ensure that patient and family develop a reasonable degree of understanding about the nature of the condition. A not uncommon finding is guilt in family members regarding what they believe to be the etiology of a psychosis. This guilt may then be displaced and projected through the use of the hex system onto "jealous" in-laws or friends. It is important that this possibility be explored and alternative explanations offered. Sometimes because of Hispanic patients' difficulty with English there is reluctance to ask questions or seek clarification. A more aggressive approach is then required on the part of the therapist.

There have also been a number of reports in the literature of good results with group therapy with less disturbed Hispanic patients. Special problem-focused groups have been used to good advantage with groups such as pregnant adolescents. Almost all workers have stressed that in the psychotherapeutic work with Hispanics great flexibility by the therapist is important—flexibility in demands for punctuality, attendance, and other requirements. Here again, it must be remembered that Hispanics are overrepresented among the poor and have the same difficulties that all poor people have with transportation, baby-sitting, fees, and basic survival.

Pharmacotherapy has a position of importance with Hispanics. Mexican Americans at least appear to be disposed, for historical reasons, to resort to pharmacological means to alleviate suffering; Mexico during Aztec times had an extensive pharmacologically active pharmacopeia. To this day, *curanderos* (folk healers) prescribe herbs and other ingestible substances for a variety of physical and emotional maladies. Also, until recently all kinds of drugs were easily available from pharmacies in Mexico without a physician's prescription. These traditions incline Chicanos to some degree to accept pharmaceutical intervention more readily. There are also anecdotal reports[22,23] needing scientific verification that Hispanic patients have a greater intolerance to anticholinergic drug side effects and require lower doses of tricyclic antidepressants. It is possible that specific variations in drug reactivity or other physiological differences might be found with proper study.

CONCLUSION

This has not been an exhaustive review of the state of knowledge of Hispanic mental health matters. Rather, I have attempted to stimulate the reader's curiosity about Hispanics. I purposely omitted mention in the introduction about where Hispanics live in the United States in order not to reinforce the view that Cuban Americans live only in Miami, Puerto Ricans in New York, and Chicanos in Los Angeles. The reality is that Hispanics are present in large and growing numbers in unexpected places: Washington, D.C., Chicago (about 1,000,000), New Orleans, and the Midwest. My feeling is that clinicians throughout the United States are and will be seeing larger numbers of Hispanic patients. In an ideal world perhaps every minority group patient should have a like-minority group professional with whom to work, but short of this Utopia, nonminority workers need materials such as this to provide guidance and understanding in dealing with patients different from themselves.

REFERENCES

1. A. Padilla and P. Aranda, *Latino Mental Health, Bibliography and Abstracts*, Alcohol, Drug Abuse and Mental Health Administration, Washington, D. C., 1974.
2. A Padilla, E. Olmeda, E. Lopez, and R. Perez, *Hispanic Mental Health*

Bibliography II, Monograph #6, Spanish Speaking Mental Health Research Center, University of California, Los Angeles, 1978.
3. J. M. Casa and S. E. Keefe (eds.), *Family and Mental Health in the Mexican American Community*, Monograph #7, Spanish Speaking Mental Health Research Center, University of California, Los Angeles, 1978.
4. E. G. Jaco, Social factors in mental disorders in Texas, *Social Problems* 4(4):322–328, 1957.
5. D. Ramirez, *A Review of the Literature on the Underutilization of Mental Health Services by Mexican Americans: Implications for Future Research and Service Delivery*, Monograph published by Intercultural Development Research Association, San Antonio, Texas, 1980.
6. V. Abad, J. Ramos, and E. Boyce, A model for delivery of mental health services to Spanish-speaking minorities, *American Journal of Orthopsychiatry* 44:584–595, 1974.
7. C. D. Chambers, W. R. Cuskey, and A. D. Moffett, Demographic factors in opiate addiction among Mexican Americans, *Public Health Reports* 85(6):523–531, 1970
8. J. F. Maddux and D. P. Desmond, Obtaining life history information about opiod users, *American Journal of Drug and Alcohol Abuse* 1(2):181–198, 1974
9. A Morales, *Ando Sangrando*, Perspective Publishers, La Puente, California, 1972.
10. F. Kline, F. X. Acosta, W. Austin, and R. G. Johnson, The misunderstood Spanish speaking patient, *American Journal of Psychiatry* 137(12):1530–1533, 1980
11. L. R. Marcos, M. Alpert, L. Urcuyo, and M. Kesselman, The effect of interview language in the evaluation of psychopathology in Spanish-American schizophrenic patients, *American Journal of Psychiatry* 130(5):549–553, 1973.
12. H. Fabrega, Jr., A. J. Rubel, and C. A. Wallace, Working class Mexican psychiatric outpatients, *Archives of General Psychiatry* 16(6):704–712, 1967.
13. V. Abad, J. Ramos, and E. Boyce, Clinical issues in the psychiatric treatment of Puerto Ricans, in: *Transcultural Psychiatry: An Hispanic Perspective* (E. R. Padilla and A. Padilla, eds.), Monograph #4, Spanish Speaking Mental Health Research Center, University of California, Los Angeles, 1977.
14. R. Fernandez-Marina, The Puerto Rican syndrome: Its dynamic and cultural determinants, *Psychiatry* 24(1):79–82, 1961.
15. W. J. Grace, Ataque, *New York Medicine* 15:12–13, 1959.
16. D. Alegria, E. Guerra, C. Martinez, and G. Meyer, El hospital invisible: A study of curanderso, *Archives of General Psychiatry* 34(11):1354–1357, 1977.
17. C. Martinez, Curanderos: Clinical aspects, *Journal of Operational Psychiatry* 8(2):35–38, 1977.
18. E. Olmedo and S. Lopez, *Hispanic Mental Health Professionals*, Monograph

#5, Spanish Speaking Mental Health Center, University of California, Los Angeles, 1977.

19. E. Jones, Social class and psychotherapy: A critical review of research, *Psychiatry* 37(4):307–320, 1974.
20. A. Kleinman, L. Eisenberg, and B. Good, Culture, illness, and care: Clinical lessons from anthropologic and cross-cultural research, *Annals of Internal Medicine* 88(2):251–258, 1978.
21. L. Comas-Diaz, Puerto Rican espiritismo and psychotherapy, *American Journal of Orthopsychiatry* 51(4):636–645, 1981.
22. R. Fieve, Pharmacotherapy here and abroad: Differences in side effects, in: *Transcultural Psychiatry: An Hispanic Perspective* (E. R. Padilla and A. M. Padilla, eds.), Monograph #4, Spanish Speaking Mental Health Research Center, University of California, Los Angeles, 1977.
23. C. Zoch, Personal communication, San Jose, Costa Rica.

4

Therapy for Asian Americans and Pacific Islanders

JOE YAMAMOTO

INTRODUCTION

Asian Americans constitute a highly diverse group of people who populate most of the planet Earth. To be asked to discuss the therapy of Asian Americans and Pacific Islanders, and to respond to such a request as if this were a feasible and thinkable undertaking, requires a bit of grandiosity. Thus, from the very beginning I have to begin with a caveat. I must acknowledge the diversity and complexity of the peoples of Asia and the Pacific Islands, and for that reason this chapter cannot pretend to outline therapy for each and every cultural subgroup. The task becomes even more monumental when one considers the generational differences, the special cases, and the individual differences that are important among all human beings regardless of ethnicity.

JOE YAMAMOTO • Neuropsychiatric Institute, University of California Medical School, Los Angeles, California 90024.

Having initiated the chapter with comments about the many nations that Asia comprises and the many diverse groups that populate the Pacific Islands, this effort will be directed at describing specific issues related to some Asian and Asian American and Pacific and Pacific American groups. Moreover, as a Japanese American, I am most familiar with the cultural issues related to the treatment of Japanese Americans.

A few publications are available dealing with the subject matter of this chapter. The National Institute of Mental Health has published a bibliographical source.(1) In addition, several faculty members of the Department of Psychiatry of the University of Hawaii have published a pioneering volume that examines issues in the treatment of Asian Americans and Pacific Islanders.(2) Thus, beginning with a paucity of information, an increasing number of contributions are being made that should be helpful in planning better services for Asian Americans and Pacific Islanders.

THE ASIAN AMERICAN AND PACIFIC ISLANDER EXPERIENCE

Historically, the immigration of Asian Americans to the United States began in the 1850s with the entry of Chinese immigrants who were brought in as a source of cheap labor for the gold mines and for work on the railroads of California. Subsequently, Asians were imported to work on plantations in Hawaii, and to serve as a labor force as needed in California and the Pacific Coast states.

The Chinese were followed by the Japanese and later by Filipinos, Koreans, and others who migrated from Asia. In Hawaii the native Hawaiians were edged out of their original landholdings, which contributed to the eventual loss of their tribal ways. Because the Hawaiians were only a small minority group, they were discriminated against, became the butt of prejudicial action of all sorts, and suffered the fate of indigenous inhabitants similar to that of the Alaskan Eskimos and American Indians. In Hawaii, however, some portions of the Hawaiian culture, including the use of pidgin English and a certain relaxed and fun-loving life-style, have been perpetuated by those who subsequently have peopled the islands.[(3)] An explicit example of this is noted in the parks, which display signs stating, "Have Fun."

In Hawaii, because Asians and Pacific Islanders constitute a majority of the population, a different social learning experience for Asian Americans and Pacific Islanders has been shaped. Asians have also been able to maintain their cultures better in Hawaii because of the more hospitable ecological and cultural atmosphere, which has resulted in often striking cultural differences when compared with their counterparts on the mainland. This is apparent in several ailments—e.g., when comparing heart disease among Japanese in Japan, Hawaii, and mainland United States (California), there is a gradient, with the lowest incidence in Japan, the next in Hawaii, and the highest in California, where the Japanese Americans have rates comparable to those of the Caucasians.[(4)]

From the 1850s through World War II, Asian Americans were the target of prejudice and discriminatory actions of all sorts. Laws related to the entry of the Chinese exemplified this in that there were laws prohibiting the immigration of wives of men already in the country. The Oriental Exclusion Act stopped immigration of all Asians after 1924.[(5)] In California and other coastal states, there wre discriminatory laws about the ownership of land (The Alien Land Act, which prohibited Asians from owning American land). Discrimination also existed in housing, employment, and educational opportunities. Fulfillment of the American dream could only be a fantasy. Compounding this, Asian Americans were stereotyped in derogatory ways—e.g., both the Chinese and Japanese have been described as sneaky and sinister at one time or another during the history of their immigration to the United States. Fortunately, these stereotypes have undergone some change over the years. After World War II this situation was improved by the civil rights movement of the 1950s and 1960s. For Asian Americans, although the situation has improved significantly, prejudice, discrimination, and racism still persist.

The targets of discrimination vary depending on geographic location and historical era. For example, before World War II, Asian Americans were discriminated against in the states of California, Oregon, and Washington. Since World War II, discrimination and prejudice have been more subtle and indirect. In contrast, even in Hawaii, which prides itself on a certain cultural tolerance and acceptance of cultural pluralism, tiny minority groups such as the Samoans suffer from discrimination.

Specifically, let us focus on the experience of the Japanese Americans just prior to, during, and following World War II. My knowledge of this experience is personal because I grew up in "Little Tokyo" in Los Angeles. The only community I knew was composed of Japanese and Japanese Americans. The elementary school that I attended was 95% Japanese. Many of the Japanese Americans also attended Japanese school in the afternoons and on Saturdays in order to learn the Japanese language and culture, along with proper Japanese manners. Before the war, despite the considerable progress of the Japanese American group, it was not unusual for college-educated Japanese Americans to have to work as gardeners and as clerks in supermarkets. Thus, occupational opportunities, including farming (the occupation of the original immigrants), were quite limited. Available only were unskilled laboring positions and small-business ownership. Middle-class positions in the majority community and civil service jobs in the ethnic community tended to be closed.

With the beginning of World War II, most of the Japanese Americans were placed in America's relocation centers.[6–8] This experience—which contrasted with the experience of the Hawaii Japanese Americans, who were never incarcerated—strongly shaped the experience and reaction of mainland Japanese Americans. The duration of the incarceration varied from approximately 1 to 3 years, or until the war ended in September 1945. Those who had jobs or acceptances to colleges could gain approval to leave the camps as early as 1943. This allowed exodus of the younger and those most able to work; however, 43,000 individuals remained in the camps until the end of the war, despite the persistent efforts of the American government to resettle the Japanese Americans. Many of these people had to be literally forced out of the camps because of their intense fear of bodily harm and also because of the inertia developed as a defense to deal with their incarceration.

Since the war, the Japanese Americans have progressed; e.g., in Hawaii, many of the middle-class positions are held by Japanese and other Asian Americans. The governor, a congressman, and two senators from Hawaii are all Asian Americans. Indeed, even in California, where the Japanese Americans and Asian Americans constitute a small minority of the population, one United States senator and two congressmen have been Japanese American. This is notable progress; however, lest it be inferred that all Japanese Americans have been able to progress as well, the reader should be assured that there are those who still suffer racism, discrimination, and prejudice. Many have succeeded, but there are

Japanese Americans who suffer from the problems of being marginal to both the Japanese American and the American culture.[9]

To summarize the Japanese American experience on the mainland, there has occurred (1) a basic level of racism that was prevalent before World War II, (2) the chaotic upheaval of the relocation center experience during the war, and (3) the subsequent gradual progress of the Japanese Americans in all areas. Throughout these negative, mixed, and positive experiences, Little Tokyo in Los Angeles and Japantown in San Francisco have been islands of ethnic identity and security against the negative attitudes of the majority Americans.

THE CHINESE EXPERIENCE

Being the pioneer Asians, the Chinese experienced the greater suffering from discriminatory acts. These include quotas, laws that prevented their bringing their wives to the United States, and laws governing miscegenation.[10] Although the Chinese, like most Asian immigrants, intended to be temporary workers in the United States, many of them became permanent immigrants. Since they could not have their wives with them, they suffered from the lack of a family life, and because of limited language capabilities, they were given lower-level jobs. Anti-Oriental racism was prevalent and also resulted in limited occupational opportunities. It was not until 1965 that the Oriental Exclusion Laws were repealed. According to Gaw,[11] there were 77,000 Chinese immigrants in the United States in 1940, but by 1970, following relaxation of the exclusion laws, the number of Chinese immigrants totaled 435,000. Since a relatively high proportion of the Chinese were recent immigrants, Chinese Americans have been able to maintain the culture of mainland China, Hong Kong, Taiwan, and other overseas areas. The language spoken comprises predominantly the Cantonese and Mandarin dialects. These have been maintained due to the frequency with which Chinese students attend Chinese language and cultural schools.

IMPACT OF THE ANTI-CHINESE LEGISLATIVE ACTS

For a penetrating and sensitive description of the scars caused by the exclusion act and other discriminatory legislation, Gaw in an excellent reference points out that the exclusion of brides made the older generation of immigrants predominantly male, and now very elderly males. He also focuses upon the new immigrants, who present their own unique problems; these include increased demands for housing, jobs, education, and other human services.(11) This is exemplified in the rapid expansion of the area called Chinatown in the center of Los Angeles. Indeed, the activities of the Chinatown Service Center have been vitally concerned with the adaptation of new immigrants, many of whom do not speak English well and need services in Cantonese or Mandarin dialects.

MENTAL HEALTH: MYTHS AND REALITIES

While Kitano and Sue have pointed out that Asians in the United States were stereotyped as being "model minorities,"(12) Gaw has noted the destructive effects of both negative and positive stereotyping.(10) Especially on the west coast, Asians have been considered model minorities with close-knit family ties and dedication to work and education, but this stereotyping has made them appear to be without problems. There are, however, innumerable problems that have been hidden from public view—e.g., among the Chinese, their characteristic need for "keeping problems within one's community" gave the appearance of self-sufficiency for a number of years.

Mental Health Needs of Chinese Americans

As is the case with Asian Americans generally, the extent of mental and emotional problems in the Chinese American communities is unknown. Although Gaw points out that there has been a tremendous increase of Chinese in state mental hospitals over the past 100 years,[(11)] this finding is difficult to interpret. Berk and Hirata[(13)] have offered some opinions about this. It is probable that the person principally at risk is the older single male. This is a direct result of the discriminatory marital and family laws, which created disproportionately high numbers of single elderly males as time progressed. The Sue and Sue MMPI study,[(14)] which evaluated Chinese and Japanese males and compared the findings with those of Caucasian males, concluded that Asians showed more symptoms than Caucasians. This may be quite correct; however, the use of the test standardized with a Caucasian population in Minnesota on an Asian American population in California would naturally pose problems. For example, we have found, on using the SCL 90R (Symptom Check List 90R),[(15)] that Asian populations score higher than Caucasians. It is apparent that for accurate cross-cultural testing, culturally appropriate norms are a necessity.[(16)]

A study by Sue and McKinney[(17)] showed that Asian Americans tended to underutilize mental health services, to be more chronically and seriously disturbed at the time of initial evaluation, and to drop out of care much more frequently. These facts are also confirmed by the studies of Tsung Yi Lin.[18]

The immigrants from China speak different dialects. Considering the fact that this creates difficulty in communication even among different generations of Chinese, it unquestionably poses problems in service delivery in this country. The older generation of immigrants were mostly from the south of China and spoke Cantonese or similar southern dialects; more recent immigrants from Taiwan predominantly speak Mandarin, which is now the standard language of China. The waves of immigrants also differ in educational backgrounds; the early Chinese immigrants have been the least well educated of all Asian immigrants. Those entering recently are in many instances better educated, while those who are second-, third-, fourth-, and fifth-generation Chinese Americans have become acculturated and are usually more American than Chinese.

DEVIANT BEHAVIOR IN CHINESE

Deprived social circumstances, the problems of crowded urban ghettos, lack of job opportunities, and a breakdown in the family traditions have resulted in the formation of some gangs in Chinatown.[11] This has been illustrated by rare incidents in San Francisco, Los Angeles, Boston, and Montreal, where outbreaks of violence by Chinese youths have caused a sensation because of the dramatic contrast with the stereotype of the imperturbable Oriental.

The suicidal behavior among elderly Chinese men in the United States is at high risk, with a rate of 27 per 100,000.[11] This is in direct contrast to mainland China, where suicide in the elderly is said to be virtually nonexistent. There are interesting sex differences in that the men tend to commit suicide by taking sleeping medication and the women hang themselves, a reversal of the usual finding in this country. Some have speculated that this is because of the cultural belief that the ghost of those who died by hanging can return to torment the living. The suicide is thus a symbolic and vengeful act. On the other hand, in first-generation Japanese in the United States, hanging is the traditional method of committing suicide for both men and women.[19] Tradition, it seems, dictates the mode of suicide.

It has been stated that schizophrenic Chinese women showed a more favorable prognosis.[20] Gaw points out that there is a paucity of data regarding the prevalence of mental disorders among the Chinese in America.[11] The need for epidemiological data for this racial group is obvious.

There is also interesting documentation of a culture-bound syndrome known as "koro" reported by Professor Yap in Hong Kong.[21] This and other syndromes are common in Hong Kong, but in 2½ years of practice in the Asian/Pacific Counseling and Treatment Center in Los Angeles, there have been no reports of any cases of such exotic syndromes. It may be that patients who exhibit this type of behavior are taken to native healers—e.g., practitioners of herbal medicine, acupuncture, and/or moxibustion. They also have the advantage of choosing healers who follow either Confucian or Buddhist teachings.

THE FILIPINO EXPERIENCE

Araneta[22] points out that Filipino immigrants vary in several ways. In contrast to Japan, whose people formed a more or less homogeneous ethnic group, the Philippines Archipelago consists of thousands of islands where many dialects are spoken, with each island having its own language and customs. Not only are there many tribes and dialects, but the people of the Philippines comprise many different ethnic groups, including Negritos, Chinese, Vietnamese, and invaders from Indonesia and the Malay Peninsula. Most of the present-day Filipinos are said by Araneta to be descended from the Indonesian and Malay groups. However, there is a long history of colonialism in the Philippines, and Araneta points out the importance of the colonial rule in introducing not only Catholicism but also dependency, comformity, and fear. Three hundred years of Spanish colonization have left their imprint on the Philippines, and American colonialism also has had an impact on the Philippines in that all educated Filipinos speak English. Ethnically, Filipinos are principally Malasian and Indonesian, but with definite Chinese, Spanish, and American influences apparent in their culture.

Despite the multiple tribes, the various ethnic derivations, and the impact of colonialism, there are certain common cultural values. These are apparent in the strong kinship ties also reflected in the spirit of mutuality and togetherness, and an expressive evidence of gratitude similar to the Japanese emphasis on reciprocity of favors. Respect and reverence of elders is emphasized, which Araneta attributes to the Chinese influence as well as to the education of the Catholic church. It is probable that Filipinos also learned the "macho" male role from the Spaniards. Furthermore, there is a supernatural orientation and an emphasis on shame; to be without shame is unacceptable in Filipino culture.

The immigration of the Filipinos to the United States has varied as with most Asian immigrants. The initial waves were imported for work on the Hawaiian sugar plantations and for cheap labor in California and Alaska. Filipinos, however, were different from other Asian immigrants; they were citizens of a U.S. territory and thus were nationals. While they were considered to have the rights and privileges of citizens, laws prevented them from voting, owing property, and intermarrying. As a result, most of the original Filipino immigrants before World War II were single laborers, almost all men.

In 1935 the Filipinos were granted independence and an immigration quota of 50 per year was imposed. Filipinos also continued to be recruited as cabin attendants in the United States Navy and could become regular noncommissioned navy personnel. Filipinos were then placed in the peculiar dilemma of having some of the rights of Americans while others were withheld because of the limitations imposed by racism and persistent discrimination.

THE FILIPINO COMMUNITY IN THE UNITED STATES

Araneta says the largest concentrations of Filipinos in the United States are in Hawaii and San Francisco. Filipino families still have more men than women (reflective of the past restrictions on immigration); the ratio of males to females is higher among the elderly who had been laborers and remained single because of federal regulations. The average size of the Filipino families may be somewhat larger than the American average. Extended kinship ties are stronger than in other American families, even including Asian American families. Among the problems of the Filipino community are the small percentage of young Filipinos enrolled in college, as contrasted to the majority of Americans, and in the very high percentage of Filipino men employed in low-skilled, low-paying jobs (40%). Because of these factors there is a reduced income level, which is a current problem for the young unskilled Filipinos as it was a problem for the elderly who were able to work only as laborers when they were younger.[20] Interestingly, problems similar to those in the United States are reflected in the Philippines, where there is a social continuum that "ranges from the very highly westernized socioeconomically advantaged group to a very traditional, unwesternized economically deprived group."[22] Amaranto[23] conducted a study of Filipinos in New York and observed the following complaints from a questionnaire survey: (1) loneliness and homesickness, (2) language difficulties, (3) work inaccessibility, (4) racial discrimination, and (5) difficulty in adjusting to the American way of life. To these he added the legislation against miscegenation and against the immigration of Filipino women, resulting, until recently, in severe unresolvable sexual frustration.

MENTAL HEALTH PROBLEMS OF FILIPINOS

The first group of immigrants were essentially from rural settings and not only had to adjust to the hard labor but also had to adapt eventually to American urban life. Another striking difference made adaptation difficult: Societal values in the Philippines emphasized dependency and membership in an extended kinship group; in contrast, in the United States strong emphasis is placed on individualism.

Since the repeal of the antimiscegenation laws, roughly one-third of the Filipinos have married interracially. Intermarriage, however, has produced some problems linked to the cultural definitions of sex roles.[22] In the Philippines women are appreciated in homemaking and child-rearing roles, while in the United States most women work outside the home. This has produced a conflict for some Filipino men, who feel somehow diminished by working wives since for them they do not meet their cultural sex-role expectations.

MENTAL HEALTH OF FILIPINO AMERICANS

Filipinos are also reluctant to seek treatment for mental disorders; this is related to Filipino conceptualizations of mental illness as well as to the feeling of shame. Araneta reports that "mental illness is viewed as a form of punishment for misdeeds of the patient or member of his family." Some Filipinos believe in spirit possession, others consider mental disorders as hereditary weakness or due to physical strain, while still others hold mental illness to be the result of sexual frustration, excesses, or unrequited love. As in Japan, the presence of the mentally ill person in the family is detrimental to the marriage prospects of other family members. When mental disorder becomes apparent, Filipinos in the Philippines turn to the family priest or a spiritual healer; this, to some degree, holds true in Filipino communities in the United States. Consonant with the cultural beliefs, a rest cure may be prescribed along with solutions for the sexual frustrations, after prayers and exorcism have been initiated; finally, medical consultation may be requested. When this does occur, it is important to establish consultation first with a recognized leader of the extended family. The social impact of the patient coming out of the family closet is an important family issue and requires that the head of the clan be consulted for his permission. Psychiatric hospitalization then is viewed as permanent and is the last recourse.

In psychotherapeutic approaches to Filipino Americans, Araneta recommends seeking counsel from the leaders and the elders, consideration of religious rituals and traditional healers, and an awareness of the importance of doing penance.

SUMMARY STATEMENT FOR ALL ASIAN AMERICANS

Legislative acts have plagued Asian Americans and other minority groups. Indeed, it was only in the last 20 years that the antimiscegenation act was repealed. Prior to that time, it was illegal for Asian Americans to marry Caucasian Americans and others. All in all, what pervaded the American culture was the myth of the melting pot, with the implication that if only one worked hard enough, persevered, obtained a good education, was clean and honest, and worshipped God, one could become an American. Of course, prior to World War II this meant a European American. This excluded the minorities—the blacks, Asians, Hispanics, and American Indians.

THE IMPORTANCE OF GENERATION

Before continuing, it is important to emphasize that there are generational differences among Asian Americans. Using Japanese Americans as an example, it is important to make explicit whether it is the first, second, third, or subsequent generations of Japanese Americans to which reference is being made. Both Gordon[24] and Kitano[25,26] have pointed out the importance of differentiating generations, and Connor[27] has shown that third-generation Japanese Americans are almost acculturated Americans. Despite the stereotypical labeling of Asian Americans as "model minorities," there is, in this country, a tremendous lack of knowledge about the mental health of Asian Americans. This is partly because of the tremendous stigma, perhaps unimagined by Americans, that is attached to mental illness by most Asian American and Pacific Islander communities. This, to an extent, accounts for the underutilization of mental health services by Asian Americans and Pacific Islanders.[28,29]

Among the Chinese on the island of Taiwan (whose cultural practices are more accessible for comparison than those of mainland China) there are, in a population of 17 million, fewer than 3,000 hospitalized psychiatric patients. Although psychiatric services are less utilized in Taiwan as compared with the use of services in the United States, it does not necessarily mean that the incidence of mental illness is less. In fact, Tsung Yi Lin,[18] in a historical and important epidemiological survey, showed that the incidence of schizophrenia was similar. Similarly, in the United States—e.g., in Los Angeles—Asian Americans utilize only 40% of their share of mental health services. This reveals a potential problem: There is an urgent need for better epidemiological knowledge of the incidence of psychosis, emotional disorder, and psychiatric problems generally among Asian Americans and Pacific Islanders.

Margaret Mead's *Coming of Age in Samoa*[30] idealized the Samoans because of their natural body habits.

> Samoan children have complete knowledge of the human body and its functions, owing to the custom of little children going unclothed, the scant clothing of adults, the habit of bathing in the sea, the use of the beach as a latrine and the lack of privacy in sexual life. They also have a vivid understanding of the nature of sex. Masturbation is an all but universal habit, beginning at the age of six or seven. There were only three girls in my group who did not masturbate. Theoretically it is discontinued with the beginning of heterosexual activity and only resumed again in periods of enforced continence. Among grown boys and girls, casual homosexual practices also supplant heterosexual activity to a certain extent. Boys masturbate in groups, but among little

> girls it is a more individualistic, secretive practice. This habit seems never to be a matter of individual discovery, one child always learning from another. The adult ban only covers the unseemliness of open indulgence.

Mead also goes on to say, "Familiarity with sex and the recognition of need of a technique to deal with sex as an art, have produced a scheme of personal relations in which there are no neurotic pictures, no frigidity, no impotence, except as a temporary result of severe illness, and a capacity for intercourse only once in a night is counted as senility." In her description of the experience of the average girl growing up in Samoa, Margaret Mead says:

> adolescence represented no period of crisis or stress, but there is instead an orderly development of a set of slowly maturing interests and activities. The girls' minds were perplexed by no conflicts, troubled by no philosophical queries, beset by no remote ambitions. To live as a girl with many lovers as long as possible and then to marry in one's own village near one's own relatives and to have many children, these were uniform and satisfying ambitions.

However, there are really no significant data about emotional health or emotional disorders among Samoans. On the island of American Samoa, with a population between 20,000 and 40,000, there are no psychiatric hospitals. No psychiatric services are available; indeed, medical facilities are very sparse. In California it is estimated that there are approximately 20,000 Samoans, most of whom live in the city of Carson; yet no one knows the incidence of emotional disorder. Pilot studies done by Yamamoto, Satele, and Fairbanks[31] showed that on the Symptom Checklist 90R, Samoans scored generally higher than American normals. However, the results of a self-administered test as a symptom checklist cannot be taken at face value until norms are available for the population in question. This would apply for Samoans in California and also for Samoans in American Samoa. Toward that end, a comparison was conducted of the SCL 90R in Samoans on the island, and again it was shown that the subjects in Carson and in Samoa, none of whom were patients, scored higher than American normals. Because of this, there is an apparent urgent need to evaluate in a more systematic and structured way the emotional health and the incidence of emotional disorder among Samoans. In an initial effort to accomplish this, a pilot study was done using Wing's Present State Examination.[32]

The study demonstrated that, of 29 (1 Tongan was inadvertently examined) Samoans examined with the Present State Examination, none was psychotic. Of those who had minimal signs of emotional symptoms, there were 10 women and 3 men. Only 1 showed signs of more than minimal social impairment. There were 2 who showed symptoms of depression. Thus, this pilot survey with the Present State Examination suggests that emotional disorder is not rampant among Samoans. We still need to understand, therefore, why they respond differently compared with American normals on the SCL 90R. The availability of the results of this study awaits a determination of the relevancy of a computer analysis utilizing a program that generates diagnostic information.

Mental Health Needs of Asian Americans

As has been noted, there is urgent need for accurate and reliable epidemiological data for the various Asian American groups.

In contrast to the general underutilization of psychiatric services by Asian Americans, it should be noted that in Japan, the development over the past 10 to 15 years of private hospitals has apparently fostered utilization, since the number of psychiatric inpatients has increased tremendously. It is estimated that approximately 320,000 psychiatric patients are currently hospitalized. In Japan, national health insurance pays for private psychiatric hospitalization, and the care is similar to that found in American stateside hospitals. In spite of low-cost inpatient care and relatively low patient fees, these hospitals are profitable. The opposite trend in the United States has resulted in decreased numbers of inpatients in psychiatric hospitals, with emphasis on community care, so that now there are only 125,000 inpatients in our nation with a population almost twice that of Japan.[33]

Utilization of mental health services by Asian Americans is partly obstructed by lack of bicultural and bilingual service. Now that these services have become available in at least one area—e.g., the Asian/Pacific Counseling and Treatment Center in Los Angeles County—the number of patients seeking care has increased enormously since its inception in 1977. The presence of clinicians who speak their language and who understand something of their cultural backgrounds is important for Asian Americans and Pacific Islanders. A study of the first 400 patients seen in a little over a year of operation revealed that many were chronically psychotic, with diagnoses of affective disorders and psychoses. The vast majority of the patients required less in the way of medication than did white American patients with comparable diagnoses. This is an important consideration for Asian Americans because the dosage of medications may have to be tailored to their specific needs.[34] It has been noted by Asian American clinicians in the United States, and also by clinicians in Japan, that patients can be maintained on lithium with serum levels lower than those recommended for white American patients.[35] The author has had the experience of treating patients who responded well clinically on levels of 0.4- to 0.5-milligram equivalents of lithium.

Many Asian American and Pacific Islanders live in the inner cities of urban centers of the United States, and consideration must be given to the deprived economic and social circumstances and the stresses of alienation of these people. As with many recent immigrants, Asians and Pacific Islanders have had difficulty with job discrimination and economic deprivation. This can result in depressive syndromes and other emotional problems, as is revealed in a study of Vietnamese (ethnically Chinese) refugees in 1975.[(36)] It was found that the refugees, although stressed about their relatives remaining behind in Vietnam and concerned about adapting to a new culture, were mainly depressed when the head of the household did not have a job. There was a direct correlation between the level of depression on the Zung Depression Scale and unemployment of the head of household. When these families were followed up a year later, most of the heads of household were employed and the occupational and emotional situation seemed brighter for the majority of the families.

Because of the close-knit families in most Asian and Pacific Islander cultures, it is necessary to examine the consequences of this closeness as it relates to mental health, and specifically for the patient who has schizophrenia or an affective disorder. Brown, Birely, and Wing[(37)] and Vaughn and Leff[(38)] have shown in Britain that highly emotional families may be an adverse factor for the health of the schizophrenic patient. Vaughn and Leff have also pointed out that there is some evidence that highly emotional families may also be detrimental for patients with depression. Of immediate concern is the extent to which the families of schizophrenic and affectively disordered patients are highly emotional and, in addition, overly critical, intrusive, and/or overinvolved. This also has been true for patients in the counseling center, and it has been necessary to try to tailor the social environment for their welfare and well-being; placement in a day treatment center is an example of such engineering. It has been demonstrated that when patients spend 40 hours or more away from highly emotional relatives, they are not as adversely affected.

There is a need for alternative care which will avoid the stigma of mental illness labeling, and which is more acceptable to Asian Americans and Pacific Islanders in contrast to what is generally available. Foster care in the community, with control of the level of adverse influence by highly emotional families, has been a useful addition. Besides, Asians and Pacific Islanders are fortunate in that more often their families remain involved with the patient, so that when the family members are not highly emotional, they can be of positive benefit in providing an adequate social environment for the patient. After the emotional state of the family has been determined and it is found that they are concerned and supportive, it is useful and highly recommended that they be involved in the discussion of the treatment plans and objectives.

In summarizing the most important aspects of treatment for Asian Americans and Pacific Islanders, therapists must keep in mind the importance of family ties, assess the strengths and weaknesses of the family, evaluate their sources of support, and, contrarily, be alert to tendencies of the family to be critical, overinvolved, and overintrusive. In addition, there is a need to be aware that Asian Americans and Pacific Islanders, as they acculturate, become more and more like all Americans. In their struggle for independence as a part of acculturation, they either may want their families involved or may prefer to have treatment planned in isolation. This issue requires evaluation, and it is important to know that for the unacculturated Asian Americans, one should *not* use the model normally prevalent for white American patients who are individualists and often live alone.

In conceptualizing the psychotherapeutic roles for the patient and the therapist, it must be remembered that in many of the Asian cultures the doctor is considered an authority. There are many implications related to the teachings of Confucious, who said, "It is important that the children be properly respectful to their parents." Thus, the patient arrives with certain expectations of the therapist: that the therapist will be a parental person, involved and concerned about the patient's welfare and actively doing things that will be beneficial. The patient in turn will be passive, respectful, and obedient.

Thus, an American democratic view of family relationships and/or therapist–patient relationship may be inappropriate for Asian patients. In addition, there may be demands for a more than usual amount of empathy, e.g., in Japanese culture it is assumed that one will try to put one's self in the other person's shoes and understand what the other person needs in the way of help. A brief anecdote can better explain this important bit of cultural behavior. During a recent visit in Seoul, Korea, the author and others were entertained by a distinguished Korean professor. Assuming that a Japanese dinner would better suit his guests' taste (Korean food is very spicy), he took us to a restaurant that served Japanese food and ordered a variety of Japanese dishes (more than enough to satisfy our needs and appetite). In Japan and Korea it is assumed that one will try to empathize with the other and put himself in the other's shoes and anticipate his needs. If you accept this and do your best to be empathic, this will be an important part of the initial psychotherapeutic relationship.

The therapist must be aware that it is possible to overly identify and empathize with the patient and the patient's family. The author recalls an Asian psychiatrist who practiced in the center of an Asian community and did everything possible to be helpful and useful to his patients and their families. In some instances, this included measures that would have been considered excessive, as, for example, administering somatic treatment in the home of patients who refused to be hospitalized. In another instance, an Asian trainee was attempting to treat a very hostile, aggressive, and dangerous paranoid patient at home, hoping that his visits on a daily basis would resolve the tremendous hostility and danger of suicide that was imminent. The trainee had to be told to arrange for psychiatric examination for hospitalization of the patient.

A final example of overextension of one's self almost had a disastrous ending. In trying to be empathic and helpful, a mental health professional made a home visit alone. This was done despite the fact that the usual procedure was that for home visits, two professional staff members are always involved. On the day of the appointed visit, however, the community worker who was to accompany the professional was ill and not available, and the latter made a judgment that it was acceptable to visit by herself. She was trapped in the apartment of an acutely paranoid, physically menacing patient who choked her—a most frightening experience.

To summarize, in the psychotherapist's role with Asian American and Pacific Islander patients, empathy of a very active and seeking sort is most important; this is what a good Asian parent does for a child. On the other hand, there is the danger of overidentifying one's self and doing things that are inappropriate or antitherapeutic; there are limits to what can be done in terms of good clinical judgment.

VARIATIONS ACCORDING TO ETHNICITY

For simplicity and brevity, it was necessary in this chapter to generalize procedures and methods that, while helpful, contribute to the danger that different ethnic groups will be stereotyped together. Several important differences are noted below. Samoans, although seen in the Asian Pacific Islander setting, constitute a quite different ethnic group (compared to Asians) with a strong tradition of extended family ties, communal property, leadership by the principal chief of the village, and strong influence of the Protestant minister (most Samoans are Protestant Christians). They are a vital, natural, and seemingly easygoing people, but in this country they exhibit high rates of hypertension. They also have a high unemployment rate and are exposed to more than the average discrimination. Although they have been exposed to both British and American missionaries and education in English, many still feel more comfortable speaking the Samoan language. This language is very specific so that everything is described in a very concrete way. It was noted during a recent study with the Present State Examination that certain questions could not be asked as per the examination schedule. The Samoans tended to misunderstand unless very specific examples were given, such as, instead of the PSE question "How confident do you feel in yourself: e.g., in talking to others or managing relations with other people?" it was helpful to substitute such questions as "When you meet new people, is it quite easy for you to begin talking with them? Is shyness a problem for you?" Another question frequently misunderstood was "What is your opinion of yourself compared with other people: do you feel better, or not as good, or about the same as most?" The Samoan subjects were reluctant to admit they were either as good as, or even better than, others. This might be interpreted falsely as poor self-image or self-depreciation. A form of questioning such as "Do you like yourself?" or "Do you feel okay about yourself as a person?" usually was preferable.

Filipinos need very specific outreach efforts. Despite the presence of an excellent psychiatric social worker on the staff of the Asian/Pacific Counseling and Treatment Center, the number of applicants for clinic services has not been commensurate with the very large population in the catchment area surrounding the center. Because of this, the social worker has had to become active in taking services into the community—

e.g., providing services to the elderly in the senior citizen centers, emphasizing health-promoting behaviors and the relief of tension, or helping with the control of hypertension. Contact with people in the community in this way can help remove the stigma of seeking mental health services.

The Japanese have been in Los Angeles almost as long as any of the Asian groups. Because of this, and the recent relatively lower immigration rate, the number of acculturated, English-speaking patients is higher in this group than among recent immigrant groups such as the Vietnamese, Koreans, and other Indochinese refugees. This contrasts with the language limitations of the early generation of Japanese immigrants. Nevertheless, for all of these groups, it is important to have a welcoming atmosphere. Toward this end, the staff should all be bilingual and bicultural. Although the receptionist may not speak the language of the patient who appears at the appointed time, the atmosphere is Asian and welcoming. There are telephones at the Asian/Pacific Counseling and Treatment Center that are designated for the use of patients who speak only certain languages; e.g., there are separate Chinese, Japanese, Korean, Samoan, Filipino, and Vietnamese lines. These lines are also connected to answering machines to which are attached brief messages in the language spoken by the particular patient population.

DIFFERENCE OF THE GENERATIONS OF ASIANS AND PACIFIC ISLANDERS

There are vast differences between the immigrants who are recent arrivals in the United States and those that have been here for decades. Many of the more recently arrived Asians and a number of the older ones live or have lived in Asian ghettos all of their lives in the United States, have not learned to speak English, and are relatively unacculturated.

Acculturation is more apparent as the generations change, and acculturated Asian Americans may be similar to Americans in their values. Connor[27] has shown that third-generation Japanese Americans are more like white Americans in their values than they are like Japanese. This is illustrated in the frequent tendency to marry outside of the ethnic group in acculturated populations, quite in contrast with the practice of new immigrants and unacculturated Asians, who marry within their specific ethnic groups. Another example is that the rate of divorce among acculturated Asian Americans is fairly comparable to the rate of divorce among white Americans. Despite many similarities, however, Asian Americans, even when acculturated, tend to use mental health services less than do white Americans. This is apparent in the published figures in Hawaii by Kinzie,[28] in Seattle by Sue and McKinney,[17] and in Los Angeles by Mochizuki.[29] Connor[27] has shown that despite the acculturation of third-generation Japanese Americans, family ties tend to be closer among them as compared to white Americans. This may account for why a stigma is attached to mental illness and why it brings shame to the entire family, as is the case in the traditional and unacculturated Japanese families.

Tests, Rating Scales, and Interview Schedules

Very special techniques of diagnosis and treatment must be designed for unacculturated Asians. At the Asian Center, tests are available in languages befitting the cultural group. Utilized are the SCL 90R, the MMPI, the Diagnostic Interview Schedule, the Psychiatric Status Schedule, and the Zung Depression Schedule.[38–42] From the time of the opening of the center, attempts were made to orient patients to the services offered. Toward this end, Samuel Lo, Ph.D., director of research at the center, has improvised an audiovisual explanation of the services available, the personnel attending, and the potential benefits from treatment. At present, the introduction is in Chinese (Cantonese and Mandarin), and work is under way to create similar materials for each of the ethnic groups served. Other audiovisual programs planned include educational materials describing the indications for psychotherapeutic drugs, and their potential benefits, side effects, and possible complications and dangers. Since our patients may not understand English, this information is needed in their own respective languages. Center personnel are aware, however, that Asian patients may not want to listen to such information and sometimes de-emphasize informed consent. Nevertheless, it is important to make sure that each patient has an adequate opportunity to be informed. Despite these efforts, experience with the use of informed consent for investigative studies has revealed that well-meaning consent forms with specific language and inclusion of details may cause adverse reactions. Many patients have looked at the forms and declined to sign, yet have agreeably participated in evaluation and treatment.

Test materials found useful in the evaluation and diagnosis of Asian and Pacific Islander patients include the following:

1. The Psychiatric Status Schedule in Chinese, Japanese, Korean, Samoan, Filipino, and Vietnamese. Audiovisual versions are equally helpful, and the center has developed them in Chinese, Japanese, and Korean. The Chinese version is in both Cantonese and Mandarin dialects.
2. The MMPI in Chinese, Japanese, and Korean.
3. The SCL 90R in six languages.
4. The Zung Depression Scale in nine languages, including Cambodian, Lao, and Hmong.
5. The Diagnostic Interview Schedule, a new schedule,

which focuses on inclusion and exclusion criteria for DSM-III and Research Diagnostic Criteria III currently is being translated into Chinese, Japanese, and Korean.

Data on normal populations of Samoans, Koreans, and Chinese with the SCL 90R are now available. It has been observed at the center that the Asian population and Pacific Islanders all score higher as compared with normal American subjects. While a detailed analysis of the reasons is not yet available, it is important to realize that it is not appropriate to use American norms for these scales and tests. In the Cross National MMPI[43] it was found that in Japan the normal population scores 2 standard deviations above the American normal population on the depression scale. It is important to be able to use these rating scales, tests, and interview schedules, but considerable work is required to delineate how best to utilize them with patients from a different cultural background.

ALTERNATIVE SERVICES

Because of the high stigma of mental illness in Asian and Pacific Islander communities, treatment within the community and in alternative care services is vital. Only in this way will some individuals be adequately treated. The average patient tends to be chronically ill, and many of the patients seen at the Asian/Pacific Counseling and Treatment Center have been sick for 5 to 10 years. It is only when the psychosis erupts into socially undesirable behavior that the patient is brought for professional attention. If the patient could be seen in an alternative care setting, such as a specific board and care home with some professional support, then people who react adversely to highly emotional families might be placed in such settings without the stigma of mental illness labeling that results from mental hospitalization. Additional advantages are that the family can continue its close family ties without disruption, and at the same time it eliminates for the patient at least 40 hours a week of exposure to a highly charged atmosphere.

In the chronic phase of mental ililness, it is generally considered feasible to have caretakers who are not mental health professionals who can by and large assist in the establishment or reestablishment of social skills, coping behavior, and increased interpersonal effectiveness. Wing's[44] wise advice that the chronic mentally ill need to be taught how to function with their disability is certainly applicable for this group of patients.

REHABILITATION SERVICES FOR ASIANS AND PACIFIC ISLANDERS

In the work at the Asian/Pacific Counseling and Treatment Center, there has been a close liaison with the Asian rehabilitation services. This is a private, nonprofit community agency that specializes in the rehabilitation of Asian Americans and Pacific Islanders. The past emphasis of this agency has been with the physically ill, but it now includes the mentally ill. One of the shortcomings of rehabilitation programs is the too often prevalent demand that the patient achieve a higher level of functioning as a result of efforts of the program. These programs are effective for those who are acutely psychotic or acutely mentally ill, but chronically mentally ill patients pose a quite different problem in that they may not be capable of responding similarly. To the contrary, they may benefit from a continued program of occupational skill training, home skill training, interpersonal skill training, and similar methods.

COMMUNITY OUTREACH

In conceptualizing treatment for Asian and Pacific Islander populations, community outreach is an essential component of the services offered. Because of their reluctance to come to a defined mental health facility, some patients can only be served in community service center settings, such as the Chinatown Service Center. At this center, mental health professionals regularly consult with the staff and also see individuals who may be potentially emotionally disturbed. Should they require treatment, an effort is often made to have them enter the Asian/Pacific Counseling and Treatment Center. If resistance is such that they refuse to go, staff members have been advised to simply treat patients wherever they are. An excellent example of outreach activity is the work of the Korean Mental Health Task Force. This group receives federal, state, and county funds and has as its function helping recent Korean immigrants with the task of coping with the new American culture. Their staff is trained in disciplines other than mental health but is provided valuable assistance by a consulting Korean psychiatrist. A similar kind of outreach service is offered to new arrivals from the Indochinese countries by community workers supervised by a Vietnamese-speaking social worker.

Japanese mental health workers provide services to a Japanese retirement home and a community low-income apartment project, and they consult with various community agencies. They attend the meetings of the consortium of Japanese agencies and professionals delivering services to Japanese Americans.

A Filipino psychiatric social worker has done a heroic job in trying to desensitize the Filipino community about mental illness. She has initiated programs that have had a positive impact in encouraging constructive health behaviors such as dieting, stopping smoking, and relieving tension through relaxation techniques. In addition, she has been a visible part of the services offered to elderly Filipinos. Thus, although the number of defined patients has not increased dramatically, significant services are being offered in a way that is acceptable in the community.

CAMPAIGNS TO IMPROVE ACCEPTABILITY OF SERVICES

Because of the high stigma of mental health services in the Asian and Pacific Islander communities, repeated campaigns have been implemented to emphasize health-seeking behaviors—for example, relaxation training for reduction of high blood pressure, biofeedback for relief of tensions, and acupuncture as an adjunct to regular Western psychotherapeutic methods. Since we exist in the Western society and our patients are from Asian nations, we offer acupuncture along with therapy. We are planning a controlled research project examining its utility as an adjunct to psychotherapy for the treatment of depression. We also will investigate the effect of offering culturally syntonic treatment on utilization of services.

RESEARCH IN ASIAN AND PACIFIC ISLANDER POPULATIONS

In the foregoing material, some of the research done in American Samoa and in the Samoan community in Carson, California, has been outlined. Ongoing research is being conducted comparing the results of standard schedules, including the Psychiatric Status Schedule, the MMPI, SCL 90R, in populations in Taipei, Taiwan, with the collaboration of Prof. Eng-Kung Yeh. One hundred Taiwanese outpatients have been examined and will be compared with 100 outpatients in the walk-in clinic at UCLA Neuropsychiatric Institute. Collected data will include clinical diagnoses of patients in both settings and computer printouts of the responses on 320 questions related to the mental status examination. This will allow comparison of patterns of symptoms for a variety of mental illnesses in both settings. We hypothesize that a much higher percentage of patients in Taiwan will be psychotic (and probably chronically psychotic) because of the stigma of mental illness in Taiwan, the relative acceptance of psychotic individuals in the community, and the reluctance to use mental health professionals except in urgent situations that require social control, hospital admission, or other measures.

THE USE OF NATIVE HEALERS AND INDIGENOUS METHODS

In the United States, there has been a long and honorable tradition of native healers. One case history of a young Navajo Indian illustrates this. In trying to help the patient, age 16, with a history of conversion seizures, a noble but unsuccessful attempt was made at using Western psychotherapeutic methods. He was seen by a very capable young medical student on a weekly basis. The results were not positive after 6 months. The Navajo medicine man had done better for this patient.

In Taiwan, where the Chinese and the Taiwanese have used native healers for centuries, it has been shown by Kleinman, Eisenberg, and Good[45] that the healers help patients with illness behaviors, whereas diseases are better treated by scientific medical practitioners. In collaborative studies in Taiwan, Kleinman has shown that many individuals use the indigenous healers for a large number of discomforts and problems in living, but this does not preclude their use of scientific medical practitioners. In many ways, however, the use of the two categories of helpers is discrete: Persons with an illness such as heart disease, tuberculosis, or cancer usually see a scientific medical practitioner. In contrast, those who have marital problems, neurotic symptoms, or depression would be more likely to seek the help of an indigenous healer or shaman.

In a recent visit to the Korean Folk Village, near Seoul, Korea, there was evidence of at least three categories of native healing in this rural setting. The Korean Folk Village had been set up as a tourist attraction, and also to maintain the history of the Korean experience. In the village, there were practitioners who told fortunes by reading palms, and it appeared that astrologers were also present. A third type of native healer were those who practiced herbal medicine. They cultivated selected plants, which became the basis for their herbal remedies. A very popular manifestation of this historical practice is in the use of ginseng for popular remedies of all sorts. In the history of China (and also in the history of medicine in Japan, because of centuries of Chinese influence), acupuncture has been an important form of native treatment. As we are all aware, acupuncture has been used for treatment of many conditions in the People's Republic of China. Before his death, Chairman Mao Tse-Tung decided that Western medicine and Chinese traditional medicine must be combined for the benefit of the people. Prof. C. I. Wu[46] described the treatment of psychotic patients in Peking with a combination of Western psychotropic medications and acupuncture. He seemed to be convinced that this method improved therapeutic results and was superior to the use of the psychotropic medications alone. Even in America, it has been reported that some schizophrenic patients respond positively to acupuncture. In addition, moxibustion has remained an acceptable and accepted form of treatment in China and Japan. Mogusa is a dried grass, which, when burned on the skin or on the needle, either simply causes heat or, in the most extreme form of treatment, can cause a scar because of the burning of the grass upon the skin. These treatments are performed on points comparable to the points selected by acupuncturists. The practices of acupuncture and moxibustion appear to be interrelated in that both of these forms of treatment involve a "laying on of the hands," and both appear to make sense to patients who believe there's something wrong with their bodies. It has been shown in many studies that somatization and the attributing of emotional problems to bodily dysfunction are very common in Asia. Psychological-mindedness and attribution of the symptoms of interpersonal conflicts is much less frequently accepted.

SUMMARY

The review of some of the case histories and cultural issues related to Asian Americans and Pacific Islanders is in an attempt to give something of the flavor of these peoples. Guam also is a territory of the United States, but we do not have a Guamian case history. Although case histories from six ethnic groups—the Chinese, Filipinos, Japanese, Koreans, Samoans, and Vietnamese—are presented, neither all of Asia nor all of the Pacific Islands are covered. Emphasized are the importance of ethnicity, acculturation, cultural issues, and flexibility in psychiatric treatment. The flexibility varies from almost standard consideration of the family as a unit versus the individual as among acculturated Americans, to reduced dosages of psychotropic medications, modified techniques for nonverbally oriented patients, adoption of authority roles consonant with the Confucian backgrounds of many Asian Americans, and awareness of the importance of empathy in various Asian cultures.

THERAPY WITH FILIPINO PATIENTS

The patients seeking treatment at the Asian Clinic represent a young population. Most of the patients were women; there were only 2 males, a young man in his 20s and one who was almost 20. The educational level of this group is higher than the average, since all have completed high school, and 5 had completed either college or training as nurses. We are aware of the underutilization of the Asian Clinic by the Filipino population, since only 37 of the 547 patients seen at the time of this writing were Filipino. Considering the population estimates, over 100 patients would have been anticipated. (The population estimates may be erroneous. The census of 1980 should clarify the number of Filipinos in the Los Angeles area.) We have assumed, however, that there are approximately 100,000 Filipinos in Los Angeles.

An interesting paper by Yolanda Mationg(47) addresses Filipino characteristics. She mentions the importance of the spirit of togetherness (Bayanihan). This may depend on what part of the Philippine Islands the Filipino is from (this may similarly vary in first-generation Japanese immigrants dependent upon their province). Family loyalties are very important in the Filipino culture: "Family interests are more important than the individual's own interests." Shame (hiya) is also important and often controls behavior since the Filipinos are taught not to do anything that might bring shame to the family. Because of the concern about bringing shame upon one's self and one's family, there is a tendency to talk about a problem as being a friend's problem. Further, there are tendencies to learn to be extra nice (pake kisama), to be compliant with the group values, and to inhibit self-expression. There is in the Filipino culture an emphasis on reciprocity (etane no loob); i.e., it is important to pay back one's obligations. Not to do so will bring shame to one's self and the family. The importance of group identity and group feelings tends to make it difficult to be a competitive individual, and there is an acceptance of, or "resignation to one's fate" (bahala na). "More emphasis is placed on adequacy rather than on excellence."

Hospitality is very important in the Filipino culture, and because of the group orientation there is less concern about individual privacy. Finally, Mationg mentions that the consequence of colonization in the Philippines by the Spaniards and the United States has resulted in characteristics that include (1) lack of organization (that is to say, participation in groups that are formally organized, such as the provincial organization in the Japanese group or the clan organization in the Chinese groups); (2) subservience; (3) nonconfrontive approach to problem solving; and (4) overorganizing (this is a present tendency to compensate for the previous lack of organization in the past).

> *Filipino Case History:* This is a young single woman almost 30 years of age who has been unemployed and living with her parents. The presenting complaint was that she is very erratic at home—she suddenly becomes sullen and angry, yells profanities, and at times locks herself in her room and cries. She appears to be talking to someone, "God," when alone in her room. She expresses a desire to kill herself and actually went to look for a knife to accomplish this, but denied her behavior when confronted later. "I'm acting strange. My mother thinks I'm crazy because I cry. The reason I cry is because

I have a toothache, stomachache, and headache." Although there is no previous psychiatric history, the patient has had problems for 2 years.

Mental status examination revealed an alert, well-oriented patient. She sat rigidly upright on the edge of her chair. Speech and movements were jerky and acclerated. Her round eyes blinked in an owllike fashion and breathing was heavy. Her affect was blunted, and associations, when she did talk freely, seemed to be loose. When she was asked direct questions, her responses seemed to be appropriate, but she tended to string words together in the middle of a sentence—for example, "love, happiness, emotions." At times the words were less well related. It is noted that she seemed somewhat grandiose and described how she earned 70,000 pesos in four months just prior to coming to the United States, selling cosmetics in the Phillipines. This is the equivalent of $9,000 and highly improbable.

Diagnostic impression was of a psychotic depressive reaction.

Treatment plans included antidepressant medications and weekly individual supportive psychotherapy, together with counseling of the mother to assist in coping with the situation.

Comments: Close family ties and the fact that a single 30-year-old lives with the family is not unusual. This case illustrates the reluctance of Asians to seek professional help; the patient was seen only after 2 years of having had symptoms.

THERAPY WITH KOREAN PATIENTS

The Koreans had very limited emigration to the United States prior to World War II. Subsequent to the Korean War and especially with the repeal of the Oriental Exclusion Act in 1965, there have been rapid increases in the number of immigrants from Korea. In contrast to past Asian immigrants, and much like the more recent wave of Filipino residents in the United States, the present group of Korean immigrants is much better educated. That is not to say that there are not uneducated or less affluent Korean immigrants; however, there is a noticeable percentage of middle-class and even affluent persons entering the country. The culture of Korea has been very strongly influenced by the culture of China, and in turn, the Koreans have influenced the culture of Japan. Thus, there have been cross-cultural influences among the three nations, with some emphasis on Confucian principles, which includes respect for the elderly, filial piety, and emphasis on the family. However, despite the cross-cultural influences, the people of Korea have maintained a distinct national identity. They view themselves as the "Irishmen of the Orient."[48] They say that the Koreans are more outgoing, friendly, and expressive of emotions than are the Chinese and the Japanese.

During a recent visit to Taegu, Korea, we were intrigued by the story of how 100 years ago Korean parents used to arrange marriages for their offspring. Typically, a 12-year-old girl would be married to an 8-year-old boy. Upon hearing this, our son said, "That's unusual." My retort was, "Not in Korea 100 years ago." In a Confucian nation, one wonders what the consequences of such a traditional marriage of an older girl to a young boy would be. With the Confucian emphasis on age, sex, and male dominance, it raises many interesting questions.

In the experience at our Asian/Pacific Counseling and Treatment Center, a very high percentage of the Korean patients either speak only Korean or prefer to have therapy in the Korean language.

Korean Case History: A middle-class married Korean man in his mid-40s had problems with his Caucasian wife. He had migrated to the United States and married his wife over 10 years ago. The presenting problem was of marital maladjustment. As presented by the couple who were seen for conjoint and individual therapy, they described the problems as related to the man's physical abuse of his wife and his frequent emotional outbursts. Another problem was that he left home with increasing frequency, often for a day or more, but sometimes for as much as 11 days. Each demanded affection, emotional support, and help from the other, and both found that these were not being supplied. A current source of conflict between the spouses was the arrival of the man's mother, who did not speak English and who sided with him (this would be culturally expected).

It was observed early in conjoint therapy that the couple tried to get the therapist to make decisions for them. When the couple was confronted with the fact that the therapist's role was to help communicate and clarify, they stopped attending the therapy sessions.

The mother had been relocated within the Korean community away from home during the crisis. Gradually the patient became angrier at his wife and blamed her for running his life; he subsequently left the family to live with the mother.

Discussion: Although this man was a long-time resident of the United States with over two decades of American experience, had received an extensive education in the United States, had married a white American woman, and had children, he seemed to have maintained the Korean sense of identity and self-worth. His traditional value orientation included the attitude of filial piety and respect owed to his mother by his wife. It was speculated that the American wife's not understanding this, and her rejection of the non-English-speaking mother-in-law, was a substantial problem in the marriage situation.

Comments: This is an interesting case involving interracial marriage. Since the man was from Korea, the cultural conflicts in the marriage situation are paramount. The incompatibility of the Korean Confucian attitude about parents, the elderly, etc., with American individualistic values is quite apparent. The lack of acceptance of American psychotherapy despite his more than average educational background can be understood in the light of the traditional view in Korea that family problems should be managed within the family. When care is sought outside of the family, usually the patient's expectations include not only improved communications and clarification of problems but also concrete assistance and recommendations.

THERAPY WITH JAPANESE PATIENTS

The Japanese in the United States, together with the Chinese, have had several generations of American experience. Thus, the questions of generation, social class, geographical area, and other issues are much more complex.

Some Japanese Americans have been able to achieve middle-class status despite the obstacles of racism, unequal opportunities, and, for the mainland Japanese, incarceration in the relocation centers. There are both elderly and young Japanese Americans covering several generations, and the differences between the first generation and those of the third and fourth generations are remarkable.

Japanese Case History: The patient is a widow in her mid-80s who had been placed in a Japanese retirement home by her family. Her presenting complaint was homesickness complicated by her almost total blindness.

Her present illness and difficulty in adjusting began 3 months ago when she was placed in a Japanese retirement home. Despite the efforts of the staff and other retirees, she had been preoccupied with her complaint of somatic difficulties, including the problems related to her almost total blindness. She seemed to be giving double messages to the staff—on the one hand clinging to them and wanting their help, on the other hand saying she shouldn't bother them. When she was helped, she responded by distancing the staff with subtle negative remarks, resulting in considerable frustration and resentment. Among her many symptoms were poor appetite, insomnia, constipation, an increased sense of incapacity in day-to-day tasks, and loneliness and sadness at being left alone in the retirement home. She felt upset about being with nonfamily people, expressed anxiety and fear about the future, and stated that she wanted to die and go to heaven soon. She had had much difficulty functioning in a group setting and as a consequence had become more withdrawn, which seemed principally related to the distress of being separated from her own family.

Past history revealed that she grew up in Japan and came to America as a bride in her 20s with her husband. She was a homemaker and had always lived with her first husband, later with her second husband, and then with her daughter and son. Past medical history was not remarkable. She had had two cataract operations, but despite this she had limited vision. She was quite perfectionistic, immature, and nervous, which is described by the Japanese term *shinkei shitsu*. Three years ago she had visited a psychiatrist because she was distressed over the loss of her older sister. Otherwise she was in robust health.

Mental status examination revealed her to be a shy,

neatly dressed elderly widow of somewhat frail appearance. She mumbled incessantly and made grunting sounds. Her hearing was normal, but she was nearly blind. There was only light perception in her right eye, and she could make out the hand of the therapist with the left. She was well oriented, and remote, recent, and immediate memory were intact. She seemed to be depressed, anxious, and agitated, and affect was labile. Associations were logical, mainly preoccupied with somatic complaints, but there was no evidence of delusions or hallucinations. She had had some suicidal ideation, without any definite plans or intent. Her intelligence and general knowledge were average. Judgment and insight were somewhat impaired.

Diagnostic impression was of a depressive reaction secondary to the loss of family support and a major change in her social environment. Since her family lived some distance away from the retirement home, family visits were not feasible. She very much wanted to see the family, to hear from them by mail or by phone, but was ambivalent about reaching out and expressing her needs for such contacts.

Treatment consisted of weekly supportive psychotherapy on an individual basis, together with antidepressant medication. In the therapeutic sessions it was productive to help her recognize her reaction to the loss of her family relationships. The therapist also visited the retirement home to discuss with the staff the nature of her handicaps. They were eager to help, and the patient and the staff members were thus again reunited as a therapeutic team. A volunteer was recruited to help her with daily tasks. In order to provide appropriate sensory stimulation to compensate for her failing eyesight, it was advised that she correspond by audiotape with the family members. This then partially substituted for the lost relationships. In addition, Japanese Homecast was recommended so that she could enjoy the FM radio entertainment. Subsequently, a blind Japanese rehabilitation counselor was introduced to the patient, not to rehabilitate but to provide an inspiring role model.

Progress in Treatment: Initially she denied her needs and her problems in adjusting to the home. She was oversensitive and had a guarded attitude, which made it difficult for her to adapt to the group living situation. Over the course of a few months, a trusting relationship was established with her. Attempts were made to help her improve her ability to communicate with the staff and other retirees and promote a more positive relationship generally. After several months her condition stabilized and she was able to behave appropriately and become more verbal. Over the course of a year she has established new relationships with greater ease and now participates in group activities.

Comments: This case illustrates the severe stress that resulted in attempting to cope with the change from a family environment to living in a group situation among strangers (tanin). The loss of a family relationship and the distress experienced in living with strangers proved to be more than she could handle by herself. Her blindness made adjustment even more difficult. Thanks to the assistance of an empathic, culturally aware therapist, the patient responded and adapted well.

THERAPY WITH CHINESE PATIENTS

The Chinese in many ways have broadly influenced the rest of Asia. If one reviews the history of the Philippines, one becomes aware of a Chinese impact. Korea and Japan also have been much influenced by China. The Taiwanese were originally from mainland China over 200 years ago and have more recently been augmented by the addition of Nationalist

Chinese. The Chinese invented and created so many things that one never ceases to marvel at their extensive list of contributions. They contributed the writing system that is used in much of Asia; they influenced the nations bordering on China with the philosophies of Confucius and the religions of Buddhism and Taoism. The Chinese also have been well known for their tolerance of mental disorder. It is only when the Chinese patient has been in some sort of social difficulty that he or she is brought for care; otherwise the patient is sequestered at home and hidden away from public view.

> *Chinese Case History:* This is a 35-year-old married Chinese male who only recently migrated to this country. He has a history of mental disturbances and was previously hospitalized.
>
> He had a white-collar job in Hong Kong but decided to come to the United States at the urging of his wife, who wanted a promising new life. After arrival he was not able to obtain employment; he had no relatives in this country, and his wife's relatives stayed away from him. He had no friends, no one to talk to, and was extremely lonely. He became suicidal and had thoughts of harming his baby daughter. It was clear that there was a crisis in facing the new adjustment of American life as an immigrant.
>
> A Chinese psychiatric social worker and a Chinese psychiatrist were assigned to work with him. He was initially seen twice a week in individual psychotherapy by a psychiatric social worker and once a week by the psychiatrist for medication. Hospitalization was avoided due to this intervention and the patient's willingness to receive help. He came to treatment sessions on time and regularly and felt that he received the kind of help he needed—i.e., seeing people to whom he could relate. A good rapport was developed between the patient and the therapists and with the Asian/Pacific Counseling and Treatment Center, which is similar to the environment

he knew in Asia—i.e., Asian atmosphere with a strong family feeling.

The patient's wife was also involved in the treatment process, and concrete help to the family in addition to psychotherapy was provided. These included authorization of child care expenses to take care of their baby daughter, information about community resources for employment and social activities at Chinatown Service Center, and referral to State Vocational Rehabilitation Services.

After approximately 6 weeks of crisis intervention, the patient stabilized. He was more cheerful, less tremulous, better dressed and groomed, and no longer suicidal. In view of his history of manic-depressive illness, lithium carbonate was prescribed to maintain his blood level to within the normal range for Asians (which is lower than that for Americans).

The patient continues to receive treatment at the Pacific Center but on a less intensive basis. When last seen he was being evaluated by the State Department of Vocational Rehabilitation.

Comments: This is a Chinese immigrant who illustrates a frequent problem seen in patients from China: the problem of adaptation to a new culture. His second major problem is that of chronic mental illness and previous hospitalization, which anteceded his entry into this country. There is a strong probability that in a traditional mental health setting, his bipolar illness would have been treated with little attention to the cultural aspects of his suffering.

THERAPY WITH VIETNAMESE PATIENTS

Several years ago, the Vietnamese people experienced the tragedy of the loss of their nation. In the wake of the defeat of the United States forces in Vietnam and their precipitous departure from Saigon, many Vietnamese also became refugees to the United States. Thousands came to Camp Pendleton and other camps hastily set up to process their entry into the United States. It was a tragedy for the Vietnamese people for not only did they lose their land, their homes, and their jobs, but many of them were also separated from their families or lost family members in the process of escape.

Vietnamese Case History: This is a 20-year-old single Vietnamese man who was brought by his parents and older sister with complaints that symptoms he had experienced earlier had returned. These included severe social withdrawal, a lack of communication with the family members, and mumbling and smiling to himself. There were in addition severe disturbance in sleep and loss of appetite.

He had been hospitalized previously for these complaints in another state. The parents noticed their reappearance after moving to Southern California. Two months later he was brought for his first interview at the Asian Clinic. The delay was due to the fact that the family was not sure where services were available. In addition, because the symptoms were somewhat milder than before, they hesitated, hoping they would diminish and go away. But when it became increasingly clear that they would not, and when he began to disrupt the family's life, they made inquiries about where he could be referred. A family friend familiar with the clinic suggested the referral.

The whole family stepped into the office as the patient was invited to enter the therapy room. It was his mother who provided most of the background information and offered her interpretation of the causes of her son's behavior. They called it a neurological sickness, perhaps because of his refusal to wear warm clothing during winter. They also speculated it was because he had been frightened by a black student. According to the parents he had an older sister. He was the second child, but the firstborn son, of the family of 10 ranging from age 21 to 2. The parents were middle class and owned an average-size store in Vietnam, which the father managed while the mother functioned as a housewife.

The patient had been an average student in junior high school and helped his father in his free time with errands. He had very few friends. His mother described him as a good and dutiful son who was expected to carry on the family's heritage and provide honor to the family name, or at least to follow in his father's footsteps. The entire family made their escape to the United States in April of 1975 in the last days before the fall of Saigon. After several months spent in the refugee camp, they were settled in the middle west of the United States.

The patient's father obtained a factory job while the patient and his siblings attended school. He was in the ninth grade and doing well, earning A's and B's with a few C's, but 2 years later his symptoms made their appearance; his parents were too busy coping with their new environment and did not notice. Even if they did, they would probably have attributed them to his physical troubles and/or the strangeness of the surroundings.

In retrospect, the parents recounted that he would come home from school using back alleys instead of the main street, and in the middle of winter with subzero cold he would refuse to wear warm clothing, claiming that he felt warm enough. He and his parents emphatically denied that he ever used drugs. When he refused to go to school altogether he was hospitalized. He stayed in the hospital for 2 weeks and was discharged to a care camp for adolescents for 2 months and finally returned to his family much improved.

Very soon thereafter the whole family moved to the

Los Angeles area to be near relatives and to get away from the cold weather of the Midwest. They were not very informative about the first hospitalization and treatment given.

The mental status examination revealed an unconcerned, boyish-appearing adolescent of short height and average weight. His hair was short and well combed, and his clothes were neat and clean. His speech was normal, enunciation clear, and eye contact good. He was well oriented to time, place, and people. His memory of distant and recent events appeared unimpaired. He denied any delusions or hallucinations and stated that his refusal to eat was the reason for his being seen at the clinic, but he would not say why he chose not to eat and became silent after this. His mood was even and his affect seemed to be appropriate to the content of thought. When asked why he chose not to eat, he became sullen and refused to reply further. On the other hand, during the verbal exchange he never used anything but the formal form of address, and his behavior was respectful. Even when his condition deteriorated and his posture became slack, his verbal remarks remained formal and respectful. Since the parents insisted that the patient had lost much weight due to his refusal of food and sleepless nights, he was hospitalized. At the time of hospitalization, a tentative diagnosis was made of schizophrenia; he received Haloperidol and improved in 10 days, then was referred back to the clinic for outpatient follow-up. Subsequent to the hospitalization he was seen weekly for 2 months, and improvement continued. He was accepted for vocational training, where he did well, and both he and his family thought that he was cured (except for his occasional complaint of pain in the eye), so they stopped the medication and discontinued the visits to the clinic.

Two months later he was brought back to the clinic with reports that he was acting-out and that his family was unable to handle him. He was again hospitalized and then discharged 2 weeks later; this was followed by weekly visits to the clinic and for 2 months with medication. Again his symptoms were greatly reduced, his family and the patient said that he was cured, and he again stopped coming.

The prognosis appears to be less than good. Because of the lack of understanding of the chronic nature of the illness by the family, they frequently discontinued the visits to the clinic after short periods of time. These have been followed by a recurrence of the illness, which requires acute treatment. His sisters are quite concerned and resentful of his mental illness for fear this may jeopardize their chances of marrying a suitable husband if it becomes known within the Vietnamese community that their brother is "crazy." Thus, there was some consideration that it might be best for the family to put him into the board and care home, despite the fact that this would only heighten his feeling of rejection. His sisters already refuse to share the same dishes with him for fear of catching his illness. Counseling with the family has not relieved this fear of contagion.

Comments: This case illustrates the importance of the family in the treatment of the Vietnamese patient. Although very serious attempts were made to counsel the family about the chronic nature of the condition and the need for continuing treatment, we were not successful. However, we would have been remiss in not planning to advise them of the best course of treatment. Of course, some of the symptoms are uniquely related to the change from a tropical nation to the harsh winters of the midwestern United States. When I heard the story of his not wearing outer clothes, it seemed to me that he was clinging, in his stubborn refusal to shield himself from the cold weather, to the hope that he could bask in the warmth of the Vietnamese sun. It was as if he were tenaciously hanging onto the last vestiges of his lost homeland.

THERAPY WITH SAMOANS

The Samoans have been influenced by the Americans for decades. Indeed, American Samoa is an American territory, with many of the benefits of the American culture and society but without the rights of representation. In considering the utilization of mental health services by Samoans, one must recognize the fact that there are no mental health services in American Samoa. Therefore, there is no pattern of utilization of mental health counseling, and because of this, it was our expectation that Samoans who have problems in living and emotional disorders would turn to their Protestant ministers and to the principal chiefs and other leaders of their community. This community orientation, with the emphasis on the authority of the principal chief and the Protestant ministers, is well established.

> *Samoan Case History:* This is a 38-year-old divorced man, a blue-collar worker whose presenting complaints consisted of depression and excessive use of alcohol. At the time of the initial interview he seemed despondent, his eyes were teary, and he complained of having felt depressed for 6 or 7 months. He attributed the depression to his difficult new job and problems in his relationship with his fiancee. She is a caucasian woman with two children by a previous marriage. In addition, he had been arrested for drunk driving and was to appear in court. He is divorced and has a son from a previous marriage and is currently living with his fiancee. He came to the United States 20 years ago and has been employed in the building trades. He complained about his job—the wages are low, the working conditions are poor, and the employer gives the workers alochol.
>
> It was revealed that the patient drinks a six-pack of beer each day. He began drinking at the age of 16, but during the past 3½ years he has increased this amount.

The general physician he had seen prior coming to the center had prescribed a minor tranquilizer.

Examination of his mental status showed that his appearance, dress, and demeanor were appropriate, but his motor activity was slowed and he exhibited poor eye contact. There was no evidence of bizarreness, hallucinations, or delusions. His attention span and memory were good. He did have religious delusions and made several references to past wrongdoings and guilt about this. He cried often and easily. His general knowledge was good.

Diagnostic impression was of a neurotic depressive reaction. Treatment plan was for supportive therapy and guidance to help him concerning the job situation and to try to help him with his difficulties concerning his relationship with his fiancee.

The course of treatment was erratic; the patient often missed appointments and finally self-terminated. He did not advise the therapist as to his future plans. During the time that he was seen over a period of 3 months, he seemed to have made some gains and received some support in therapy.

Comments: This patient revealed work-related problems; he also used alcohol excessively, which is more common among Samoans than in other Asian groups. He appeared to have little understanding of what could be offered him, and it is not known whether he availed himself of the usual Samoan supports—e.g., the minister—or, for that matter, if they were available in his community.

ACKNOWLEDGMENTS

Appreciation is expressed to Mr. John Hatakeyama, director of the Asian/Pacific Counseling and Treatment Center, and his staff, who contributed case histories. Among those who did so are the following: Joselyn Yap, M.S.W.; Duck Soo Hahn, M.S.W.; Rock Choe, M.D.; Desmond Fung, M.D.; Julia Lam, M.D.; Samuel Lo, Ph.D.; Kenneth Yang, M.S.W.; Que Le, M.S.W.; Sachiko Reece, R.N., M.A.; Tazuko Shibusawa, M.S.W.; Adele Satele, M.S.W.; and Reupena Samuelu, Ph.D.

REFERENCES

1. J. K. Morishima, S. Sue, L. M. Teng, N. W. S. Zane, and J. R. Cram, *Handbook of Asian American/Pacific Islander Mental Health, Volume I*, NIMH, DHEW Publication No. (ADM) 79-754, University of Washington, Department of Psychology, Seattle, 1979.
2. W. W. Tseng, J. F. McDermott, Jr., and T. W. Maretzki, (eds.), *People and Culture of Hawaii*, Department of Psychiatry, University of Hawaii School of Medicine, Honolulu, 1974.
3. A. Howard, *Ain't No Big Thing: Coping Strategies in a Hawaiian-American Community*, University Press of Hawaii, Honolulu, 1974.
4. M. G. Marmot, S. L. Syme, and A. Kagan, Epidemiologic studies of coronary heart disease and strokes in Japanese men living in Japan, Hawaii and California: Prevalence of coronary and hypertensive heart disease and associated risk factors, *American Journal of Epidemiology* 102:514–525, 1975.
5. F. K. Cheung, *Recent Advancement in Study of Asian Immigrants in the United States*, An unpublished paper for NIMH, Presented at Taipei City Psychiatric Center, Taiwan, June 1978.
6. D. Thomas, *The Salvage: Japanese American Evacuation and Resettlement*, University of California Press, Berkeley, 1952.
7. M. Weglyn, *Years of Infamy: The Untold Story of America's Concentration Camps*, William Morrow, New York, 1976.
8. M. Conrat and R. Conrat, *Executive Order 9066*, California Historical Society Special Publication No. 51, 1972.
9. H. H. L. Kitano, Japanese-American crime and delinquency, *Journal of Psychology* 66:253–263, 1967.
10. A. Gaw (ed.), *Cross-Cultural Psychiatry*, John Wright-PSG Inc., Boston, Bristol, London, 1982.
11. A. Gaw, Chinese Americans, in: *Cross-Cultural Psychiatry* (A. Gaw, ed.), John Wright-PSG Inc., Boston, Bristol, London, 1982, pp. 1–29.
12. H. H. L. Kitano and S. Sue, Model minorities, *Journal of Social Issues* 29:1–10, 1973.
13. B. B. Berk and L. C. Hirata, Mental illness among the Chinese: Myth or reality, *Journal of Social Issues* 29:149–166, 1973.
14. S. Sue and D. W. Sue, MMPI comparisons between Asian-Americans

and non-Asian students utilizing a student health psychiatric clinic, *Journal of Counseling Psychology* 21:423–427, 1974.
15. L. R. Derogatis, R. S. Lipman, and L. Covi, SCL-90: An outpatient psychiatric rating scale—Preliminary report, *Psychopharmacology Bulletin* 9(1):13–27, 1973.
16. J. Yamamoto, L. Fairbanks, B. J. Kang, S. Koretsune, S. Reece, J. Yap, S. Lo, R. Samuelu, and A. Satele, Symptom checklist 90R of normal subjects from Asian/Pacific populations, *P/AAMHRC Research Review* 2(3), 1983.
17. S. Sue and H. McKinney, Asian Americans in the community mental health care system, *American Journal of Orthopsychiatry* 45:111–118, 1975.
18. T. Y. Lin, A study of the incidence of mental disorder in Chinese and other cultures, *Psychiatry* 16:313–336, 1953.
19. J. Yamamoto, Japanese American suicides in Los Angeles, in: *Anthropology and Mental Health* (J. Westermeyer, ed.), Mouton, Hawthorne, N.Y., 1973, pp. 29–36.
20. W. H. Lo and T. Lo, A ten-year follow-up study of Chinese schizophrenics in Hong Kong, *British Journal of Psychiatry* 131:63–66, 1977.
21. P. M. Yap, Koro—A cultural bound depersonalization syndrome, *British Journal of Psychiatry* 111:43–50, 1965.
22. E. Araneta, Jr., Filipino Americans, in: *Cross-Cultural Psychiatry* (A. Gaw, ed.), John Wright-PSG Inc., Boston, Bristol, London, 1982, pp. 55–68.
23. E. A. Amaranto, *Mental Health Studies of Filipino Immigrants in New York Metropolitan Area,* Report, Asian American Mental Health Research Center, Chicago, 1978.
24. J. M. Gordon, *Assimilation in American Life,* Oxford University Press, New York, 1964.
25. H. H. L. Kitano, *Japanese Americans: The Evolution of a Subculture,* Prentice-Hall,l Englewood Cliffs, New Jersey, 1969.
26. H. H. L. Kitano, Mental illness in four cultures, *Journal of Social Psychology* 80:121–134, 1979.
27. J. Connor, *Acculturation and the Retention of an Ethnic Identity in Three Generations of Japanese Americans,* R & E Research Associates, San Francisco, 1977.
28. J. Kinzie, A summary of literature on epidemiology of mental illness in Hawaii, in: *People and Cultures in Hawaii* (W. S. Tseng, J. F. McDermott, Jr., and T. W. Maretzki (eds.), Department of Psychiatry, University of Hawaii School of Medicine, Honolulu, 1974, pp. 8–12.
29. M. Mochizuki, Discharge and units of service by ethnic origin: Fiscal year 1973–74, County of Los Angeles Mental Health Service, Research and Information Section, *E. & R. Rows and Columns* 3(11):1–15, 1975.
30. M. Mead, *Coming of Age in Samoa,* William Morrow, New York, 1928, p. 136.
31. J. Yamamoto, A. Satele, and L. Fairbanks, Samoans in California, *Psychiatric Journal of University of Ottawa* 4(4):349–352, 1979.

32. J. Yamamoto, S. Jones, and R. Samuelu, Pilot survey of Samoans with the present state examination, *American Journal of Social Psychiatry* 1(2):21–23, 1981.
33. J. Yamamoto, Japanese Americans, in: *Cross-Cultural Psychiatry* (A. Gaw, ed.), John Wright-PSG Inc., Boston, Bristol, London, 1982, pp. 31–54.
34. J. Yamamoto, D. Fung, S. Lo, and S. Reece, Psychopharmacology for Asian Americans and Pacific Islanders, *NIMH Psychopharmacology Bulletin* 15(4):29–31, 1979.
35. C. P. Chien and J. Yamamoto, Asian-American and Pacific Islander patients, in: *Effective Psychotherapy for Low-Income and Minority Patients* (F. X. Acosta, J. Yamamoto, L. A. Evans, eds.), Plenum Press, New York, 1982, pp. 117–145.
36. J. Yamamoto, J. Lan, D. Fung, F. Tan, and M. Iga, Chinese-speaking Vietnamese refugees in Los Angeles, in: *Cultural Psychiatry* (E. Foulks and R. Wintrob, eds.), Spectrum Press, New York, 1977, pp. 209–215.
37. G. W. Brown, J. L. T. Birely, and J. K. Wing, Influence of family life on the course of schizophrenic disorders: A replication, *British Journal of Psychiatry* 121:241–258, 1972.
38. C. Vaughn and J. Leff, The measurement of expressed emotion in the families of psychiatric patients, *British Journal of Social and Clinical Psychology* 15:157–165, 1976.
39. L. R. Derogatis, K. Rickels, and A. F. Rock, The SCL-90 and the MMPI: A step in the validation of a new self-report scale, *British Journal of Psychiatry* 129:280–289, 1976.
40. L. Robins, *NIMH Diagnostic Interview Schedule,* Washington University School of Medicine, St. Louis, 1979.
41. R. L. Spitzer, J. Endicott, and G. Cohen, *Psychiatric Status Schedule,* Evaluation Unit, Biometrics Research, New York State Department of Mental Hygiene, New York State Psychiatric Institute, Department of Psychiatry, Columbia University, October 1968.
42. W. W. K. Zung, A self-rating depression scale, *Archives of General Psychiatry* 12:63–70, 1965.
43. J. Butcher and P. Pancheri, *A Handbook of Cross-National MMPI Research,* University of Minnesota Press, Minneapolis, 1976.
44. J. K. Wing, *Schizophrenic,* Academic Press, London, 1978.
45. A. Kleinman, L. Eisenberg, and B. Good, Culture, illness and care: Clinical lessons from anthropologic and cross-cultural research, *Annals of Internal Medicine* 88:251–258, 1978.
46. C. I. Wu, Personal communication, 1979.
47. Y. Mationg, *The Filipino-American Community: An Assessment,* Unpublished project for the Asian American Drug Program, Los Angeles, 1979.
48. E. G. Adams, *Korea Guide,* Seoul International Tourist Publishing Co., Seoul, 1976.

5

An Integrative Approach to American Indian Mental Health

R. DALE WALKER AND ROBIN LADUE

INTRODUCTION

Contemporary American Indians face many health and social problems with established roots in North American history. Current programs designed to address the unique health needs of American Indians have undergone many difficulties, including an apparent lack of culturally relevant therapeutic approaches, a severe shortage of funding and personnel, and an uncertain administration of health policies.

The scientific literature on American Indian mental and physical health has tended to focus on specific topics such as alcoholism, suicide, and violence.[1–4] These topics are of grave

---

R. DALE WALKER • Seattle Veterans Administration Medical Center, and Department of Psychiatry and Behavioral Sciences, University of Washington, Seattle, Washington 98105. ROBIN LaDUE • Department of Psychiatry and Behavioral Sciences, University of Washington, Seattle, Washington 98105. Chapter preparation was supported in part by a grant from the National Institute of Alcoholism and Alcohol Abuse (AA04401).

concern to any professional involved with Indian health but are better understood when considered in the context of overall problems and needs of American Indian people today.

Although the literature tends to treat the Indian as a single entity, prior to contact with the white man, there were over 300 distinct tribal groups in North America, each with its own genealogy. To attempt to record a definitive volume on American Indian tribes would be a Herculean task that could reach encyclopedic proportions. This is compounded by the fact that for the most part, historical information for each tribe was preserved as stories, songs, and legends, and a few writing systems. Those writing systems that did exist were destroyed by European conquerors to promote the "civilization" of these tribal groups. The picture of Indian life in North America before 1492 rests upon word-of-mouth histories, archaeological findings, and writings of Europeans who had early contact with Indian tribes. This information may not be reliable or very complete. Despite the many differences between tribes, commonalities exist, and attempts will be made to present a general view of deviant behavior for native populations. Familiarity with the historical events that have influenced the mental health of the contemporary American Indian may lead to a better understanding of the current problems and needs.

Four separate time intervals involving historical events for Indians are identified: (1) the Precontact era, prior to 1492; (2) the Manifest Destiny era, 1492–1890; (3) the Assimilation era, 1890–1970; and (4) the era of "Indian Self-Determination," 1970 to the present. Within each of these time frames, the definitions of deviancy are explored in the context of cultural values and social historical events. The hypothesized causes, consequences, and cures of deviancy are examined from the perspectives of the different eras.[5–9] Therefore, this chapter explores historical aspects of American Indian mental health, presents problems facing the American Indian population, and suggests future directions to more adequately address these needs. These three issues are reviewed in light of traditional Indian values, beliefs, and practices.

PRECONTACT PERIOD

It is popularly held that this continent was peopled by successive waves or migrations of Asians beginning at least 20,000 years ago. Such migrations back and forth across the Bering Strait may explain the great variety of cultures, languages, and life-styles seen in the over 300 tribal groups that occupied North America. The impelling force to travel throughout North and South America by these tribal groups has always been a source of curiosity to scientists and may be an important issue in medical/psychiatric treatment today. The establishment of customs, beliefs, and behavior appears to be based upon historical tradition, tribal interactions, and situational needs. In spite of the large number of different North American tribal groups, there appears to be some consistency in the development of guidelines for living for groups of people.

The acquired roles and rules of Indian people may be viewed as a survival pact. A survival pact has been defined as a set of rules that establish a symbiotic relationship among the individual, the group, and the earth. The rules of the pact touched on all aspects of life, including marriage and social encounters, food gathering, hunting and fishing, religion, and medicine. The laws of the pact are passed from generation to generation through oral histories, songs, and legends. As long as tribes followed these rules, they survived and prospered. Deviation from these rules brought punishment consistent with the jeopardy in which the tribe was placed.

The Importance of Stories, Songs, and Legends

Because only a negligible written record was left, the study of philosophy, world view, and laws of American Indians is not an easy task. Behavior in given situations, and the consequences of misbehavior and disobediance were passed along in stories, songs, and legends. All may be considered as part of the survival pact. Some of the information contained in legends has been verified by anthropological investigations.[10–17]

To the Indians during the precontact period, most of the animals and objects in the world possessed life and/or some type of supernatural power. Among these, the coyote was often seen as a great god, possessing both animal and human qualities. The coyote was cunning, deceitful, and viewed as a "trickster." He was a rule giver and rule breaker, a creator as well as a destroyer.[10] Many other animals were described in the legends, as well as mythical monsters and ogres. While the animals in these tales could be bad or good, the mythical beasts were almost invariably evil, much the same as the "boogie men" called upon to scare today's children. Mythical monsters were often symbolic of elements of the natural world: Thunderbird carried thunder and lightning on the mountaintops, or Chinook represented the wind.[10–18] Again, these creatures were used to illustrate good and evil and the consequences of failure to follow the long-established rules. Stories, songs, and legends were developed to convey a moral or rule much like Aesop's fables or the Uncle Remus stories (thought to be based upon Cherokee folklore).

Rules of Social Morality and Interactions

The tribal structures, prior to European contact and the subsequent epidemics, centered around kin groups and included cousins, aunts, and uncles, as well as parents and siblings. The local group fulfilled a central function in ceremonies, politics, and the distribution of wealth. Within each group, individual members had defined roles in the survival pact. For instance, in the northwest coast area, human interactions assumed great complexity. Here the tribes established formal chiefdom societies, with an aristocracy and fairly rigid class levels.[14,15] Marriage was encouraged within classes, and the penalty for marriage outside of one's class could be death. These rules, and the outcomes resulting from breaking them, are often talked of in the legends of the region.[10,18,19] For example, in one tale of the Yakima region, a young chief, very wise and handsome, refused to marry. To ensure themselves that the tyee's (chief's) wisdom was continued, lesser chiefs came from all across the territory to tempt the Great Tyee with their daughters. Finally, out of desperation, the Great Tyee was forced to flee and seek help from his father, Speelyai (Coyote). Despite Speelyai's help, the tyee was continually pursued by lustful maidens and their greedy fathers. Because of their disrespect, Speelyai turned the women to stone, thus protecting the virtue of the tyee and leaving a concrete example of the penalty associated with lust and greed.[10] The consequences of marrying out of one's class were also presented in a legend from Vancouver Island. A tyee had chosen a bride for his son but the woman was unattractive. The son had fallen in love with another girl, who was very beautiful but from the wrong class. As a result of the son's disobedience, the tyee sent his son and his lover to live on the moon. As suggested by these legends, the punishment for marriage out of one's class and disobedience to one's elders was often severe.[10] The legends were tangible evidence conveyed by word of mouth down through the years to remind people of the results of wrong behavior. Information conveyed by these legends was found in many anthropological sources from other native cultures in the same time period.[14,15,18,20–22]

Not all legends concerned rewards and punishment alone. Several demonstrated the humor with which Indians approached life. An example of this was the tale of Coyote, who had lustful thoughts about beautiful women, none of whom was his wife. At one celebration, Coyote approached a woman, only to find that she was really his wife, and Coyote was caught attempting to be unfaithful.[(10)]

Based both on anecdotal information from legends and on anthropological data, an ecological model has been used to describe Indian behavior during the precontact era.[(23)] Such a model recognized the interdependence between humans and their environments, both psychological and physical, and in this regard remained consistent with tenets of a survival pact. An ecological model also stressed the cycling of resources, adaptation, and succession.

Cycling of Resources

Gleanings from both the legends and anthropological material verify the importance of the proper use of natural resources. One of the most severe of calamities that could befall a tribe was the loss of a valuable resource—e.g., salmon in the Northwest, the whales or seals in the Artic, water in the Southwest. The Coyote legends tell of Coyote removing the salmon as a punishment visited on Indian people for not properly respecting and using nature's resources.

Adaptation

Adaptation was vital if there were any changes in the environment. Specialized methods of fishing had to be developed to fit the various rivers, rules guiding proper methods of hunting were designed, and rigid laws of social behavior relating to these criteria were established. Water rations and irrigation in the Southwest shaped both community and individual behavior. All of these behaviors were a part of some form of adaptation to maintain the status and survival of the group.[23–25]

Succession

The changing of power and leadership from generation to generation and the maintenance of peace within and between tribal groups are forms of political succession. From an ecological point of view, succession also refers to the gradual changes that occur in society as the environment changes.

Religion

No systematized religious beliefs, such as the Christian Trinity, were found in the tribal groups of the Northwest. However, the survival pact included supernatural and spiritual beliefs that centered around the day-to-day issues encountered by the people of the region—e.g., their sources of food, protection from enemies.[14] Because of the symbiotic relationship of the Indian to his world, it was a natural consequence that the plants, fish, and animals played important parts in their religion and spiritual beliefs.

One of the most important creatures in the life of the Northwest Indian was the salmon. Salmon remained a mainstay of food throughout the year and were also used in trade. As a tribute to, and because of the importance of, the salmon, they were seen as supernatural beings that made the supreme sacrifice—i.e., giving up their lives in order to feed the Indian. The first Salmon Ceremony, honoring the return of the salmon for another season,[14–26] became one of the more important religious ceremonies of the year.

The importance of the salmon was also reflected in the

Coyote legends of the Northwest. In several of these legends, Coyote saved the people from starvation by teaching them to catch and/or dry salmon. In the legends of the formation of the Spokane and Palouse Falls he punished his people by taking the salmon from the rivers. The importance of salmon was reflected by the total change in life-style for the people of the river, both in the legends and in reality when this resource was lost.[10,17]

Typically the religion of tribal groups was based on the close relationship between the Indian and the important components of the world—i.e., the fish and animals. The religious beliefs and practices were part of a survival pact that taught the Indian how to best use and respect the resources found in his or her environment.

Shamanism

The shaman (often known today as a medicine person) of the Northwest was usually from the lower classes of Indian society. It was not uncommon, however, for a shaman to achieve recognition outside his or her own group. According to the beliefs of the Northwest tribal groups, all illness, both physical and psychological, was caused in two ways: (1) by object intrusion, in which an object was "magically" inserted into the body by an evil spirit or a shaman, and (2) soul loss, caused by the soul leaving the body, which resulted in a slow wasting away instead of a quick death.[27]

The duties of the shaman included determining the causes of, and curing, the illness. Shamans collected fees for their services, as do physicians of today, but the shamans also turned a portion of their fees over to the leaders of the group.[14,15,27,28] As with many other aspects of tribal life, healing was often a community function, with the shaman being the central figure and aided by assistants from the group.

Shamanism was often depicted in the legends of the Northwest, with Coyote assuming the healing role. As with a real shaman, Coyote searched for the cause of the problem, enacted the cure, and received a fee for services rendered. In one legend, the fact that Grizzly had been eating Indians was brought to Coyote's attention. Grizzly was feeling ill after consuming a large number of Indians, and Coyote offered to cure his pain but actually tricked Grizzly into chasing him across a river in which he fell and drowned. Coyote did not tell the people the truth behind Grizzly's demise but instead made himself appear as the hero. This legend contained healing and morality elements found in other legends: (1) Coyote was viewed as trickster and savior, and (2) Grizzly was viewed as evil and punishable.[13,14] Respect for shamans is also taught in the process.

Causes of Deviant Behavior

Prior to increased contact with non-Indians, there did not appear to be a theory of mental illness similar to that found in western European culture of the same era. The latter included such widely disparate hypotheses as the theory of organic damage and symptomatology (mental illness was caused by localized damage to the brain); the theory of "original sin" (humans are born inherently bad); possession by evil spirits; and mental illness caused by an underlying physical illness.[29]

The Indian theories of mental illness found in the precontact era also adhered to the concept of physical illness as the causative agent of mental illness. Behaviors that today might be described as psychotic or depressed were seen as resulting from object intrusion or soul loss. Soul loss corresponded, on the basis of the description of symptoms, to what is now termed severe depression, with lassitude, lack of activity, and a general wasting away.[28,30] Other categories of problems, such as conduct disorders and deviant behavior, were viewed in the context of disobedience and treated as such. These disorders broke the rules of the tribe and were viewed as maladaptive for both the individual and the group.

THE MANIFEST DESTINY ERA: 1492–1890

Manifest destiny is a term coined in the mid-1800s to describe the desire of many Americans to possess a country that was larger than Europe and reached from the Atlantic to the Pacific Ocean. The fact that the land was occupied by numerous Indian tribes did not deter or influence their effort. This era created immense and dramatic changes in the lives of American Indians, including the decimation of tribal populations due to epidemics, and the institution of the reservation system. Each of these factors not only had a critical impact on the culture of Indian bands but also led to an enormous loss of life. Considerable descriptive literature reviewing the life of the Indian during this period exists,[25,31] but there has been little review of the impact of these changes upon the mental and physical health of Indian groups.

Consequences of the Epidemics: 1792–1890

Prior to the epidemics, which struck native populations across the continent, the American Indian often had been described by early explorers as healthy, vigorous, and with a good knowlege of medicine and healing. The major events that changed the course of history and the lives of many Indian people were epidemics of smallpox, cholera, diphtheria, and typhoid fever, which laid waste to the tribes between 1600 and 1790.[32] The ravages of European diseases were so devastating that John Lawson, an early American historian, was led to estimate that only one-sixth of the Indians survived within 200 miles of white settlements. With each advance of white settlers came panic, violence, and ultimate decimation of Indian communities.[33] The epidemics were the first of a series of events that had complex and long-term effects on the Indian people, the consequences of which may have affected their concept of mental health.

Prior to the epidemics, each tribal member had a clear role, and the welfare of an entire tribe depended upon how well each individual role was fulfilled. Following the epidemics, the deaths of such huge numbers of Indians resulted in an almost total destruction of the symbiotic relationships between the individual and the group. Equally devastating was the loss of many of the leaders and elders of a number of tribes, which left few to teach the young the ways of survival. The epidemics also changed the role of the shaman and the definitions of illness as they were understood in the preepidemic/precontact period. It was the job of the shaman to cure all illnesses regardless of cause. When it was not possible to heal those ill with "non-Indian diseases," it changed the way the shamans were viewed by their tribes and detracted greatly from their power. A shaman who could not heal himself or his people was of little practical or spiritual value to his tribe. The weakened power of the shamans helped to pave the way for greater acceptance of European religions and medicine.[34]

Impact of the Early Explorers and Traders: The Northwest Experience

In the 1790s the Northwest was explored by sea (the Vancouver mapping and naming expedition of 1792) and by land expeditions by the fur traders in the late 1700s. With the arrival of white men, many of the tribes who had been traders for centuries saw economic possibilities for their people. Therefore, the first traders were welcomed. In 1804, following these early expeditions, Lewis and Clark made their historical journey to the Pacific and were successful in mapping parts of the Northwest. It did not take very long for word to filter back to the East of the rich and plentiful lands available in these regions.[14,15,25]

The British were the first Europeans to take advantage of the enormous resource potentials of the Northwest. Originally it was believed that they had acquired an understanding of Indian life since they interfered minimally with the Indians' hunting and fishing rights. Beginning with Thompson's expedition in 1797, however, it was found that many British traders used alcohol as a means of achieving their ends.[35] By 1812 British, American, and Russian fur companies had made their mark in the Northwest and Rocky Mountain regions by dominating the fur trade and establishing posts such as Forts Astoria and Vancouver. Perhaps the best known of these companies was the British-owned Hudson's Bay Company, which employed a variety of people—e.g., French, Canadian, Indian, British, and Polynesian. Following the defeat of the British in the War of 1812, Americans began to envision the occupation of the entire continent. Large sections of land in the central and northwest sections of the country that were occupied by Indians were left vacant due to the decimation of many tribes by diseases and epidemics. Led on by the call for westward migration, settlers found this land attractive for farming, ranching, mining, and other financially rewarding enterprises. The pattern of Indian disease, vacating of land, and white settlement that occurred earlier in the northeastern and southeastern parts of the country became universal. Not understood by the newcomers was the fact that the Indian tribes still claimed this land as ancestral property, although remaining populations were not large enough to occupy it.

As time passed, more and more Americans entered the Northwest, and the relationships between whites and Indians began to deteriorate.

Effects of the Later Epidemics

By 1825 Indian tribal population in the Northwest stabilized after the first wave of epidemics.[36] But in 1829 disaster again struck, this time in the form of "intermittent fever." The exact nature of this disease remained unknown, but it is thought to have been either malaria or pneumonia.[36] The native people, already reduced in population, were devastated by another 80% loss of life.[37] The consequences of the first epidemics were repeated, but this time no recovery in population occurred for several generations. The loss of culture, language, and religion was further enhanced by missionaries and governmental officials, who soon appeared to impose their own doctrines and restrictions.

Conversion to Christianity

Missionaries were able to exert a powerful influence over the Indian tribes. Several factors seemed to account for this occurrence. The native populations had been decimated by disease during the early contact period, causing the loss of long-standing rules for social order and behavior, economic opportunities (intertribal trading), and hunting and fishing.[29,37] The role of the shamans was altered and reduced in power within the tribe due to their inability to cure European diseases. Most of the elders and tribal leaders who taught the rules of behavior, religion, and socialization to tribal members were gone. With near total devastation and disruption of life among Indian people throughout the country, the Christian religion filled the emotional and spiritual void. Missionary work was accomplished by the Puritans in New England, the Jesuits in California, the Presbyterians in the Southeast, and the Catholics in the Southwest. It was the Jesuits who followed the fur traders into the western region and established the first Northwest mission in Toledo, Washington, in 1837. Regardless of the religious denomination, the end results of their influence was the same: conversion of the native people and a further loss of native culture.[15,25,37]

While not always a primary goal of the missionaries, the religious indoctrination helped to settle the "frontier" and ease the natives "as peacefully as possible, into oblivion."[25,38] It may seem strange that a people would embrace religions that aided in bringing about the end of their culture, but the life of the Indian was unpleasant at that time and there was little hope for a total return to the traditional ways. The Christian promise of a better afterlife must have seemed quite inviting. In addition, the rituals of Christianity provided replacements for the loss of traditional Indian ceremonies, rules for behavior, consequences of misbehavior, and spiritual leaders. Missionaries often cared very deeply for the Indians in their jurisdiction, but most failed to understand the remaining traditional values and beliefs still held by many of their converts.

Treaties and Reservations

In 1829 Andrew Jackson argued in his presidential address that the only solution to the Indian problem for the citizens of the state of Georgia was the removal of the Cherokees to an area west of the Mississippi. A similar fate soon befell the Choctaw, Creek, Seminole, and Chickasaw in what is known as the Trail of Tears. Many Eastern tribes were relocated to an area distant from a white settlement in what is now Oklahoma. In 1854, as part of the Kansas-Nebraska

Act, efforts were made to remove the Indian barrier to westward expansion, and a new Indian policy was developed in the office of the secretary of war. All Indians, including those in the Northwest, were to be confined to reservations, remote from white settlements.[35,39] Reservations were to be protected from greed and the degrading influences of whites. Indians on reservations would be governed by law and were to have the help of missionaries and teachers.[37] Vast amounts of land in the western United States were initially set aside for Indian people, but the increasing number of settlers along with many speculators led to a continuing reduction in lands and relocation of tribes. The elimination of reservations, the placement of rival bands upon the same reservation, the exiling of strong tribal leaders, and the passage of legislation making the practice of Indian language, religion, and customs illegal combined to make reservations unhappy and miserable.[12,13] The implementation of boarding schools, both by the government and by various religious groups, focused upon the removal of all traces of "Indianness" from children (language, dress, values, beliefs, religion, and customs) and their replacement with the accouterments of white civilization.[38,40] In later years, boarding schools would have "before and after" pictures to reflect their effectiveness in carrying out their tasks. Children were punished severely for speaking in their own language and concluded that to be Indian was to be bad. Many Indian children with boarding school experiences grew up with hatred toward their parents, their heritage, and themselves. Problems in contemporary Indian life such as cultural ambivalence, depression, and low self-esteem can often be traced to boarding school experiences.[41,42]

The Indian did not always accept passively the restrictions and laws imposed by the government, and many armed skirmishes were fought between whites and Indians across the country. Famous examples include the flight of the Nez Perce, led by Chief Joseph, and the Battle of the Little Big

Horn. Many other tribes fought to retain their lands: the Sioux, Yakima, Apache, and Comanche, to name a few.[43,44] After military defeat, there was a call for harsh punishment of the leaders and their tribes to ensure against future uprisings.

Revitalization Movements (pre-1890): Shakers, Dreamers, and the Ghost Dance

A reaction against their bleak life came about in the latter half of the 1800s with the emergence of several religious cults known as "revitalization movements."[45,46] Because of the loss of knowledge and culture engendered by the epidemics, as well as the influence of Christianity, the Indian religious movements may not have maintained a clear traditional picture. The "new" religions included the Shakers of the northwest coast, the Dreamers of the plateau, and the Ghost Dancers of the plains.[45–48] All contained elements of both Christian and native beliefs and practices.

Indian revitalization movements were no better understood by whites than were the older traditional tribal customs and beliefs. Laws were passed in attempts to suppress and eradicate most traditionally associated religious practices and beliefs. Even though the traditionally associated religions were influenced by Christianity, Indians were punished for what had actually been encouraged by the government, the boarding schools, and the missionaries.[45,46,49,50]

Specific Theories of Illness and Rules of Behavior

Religious movements in the 18th and 19th centuries had a profound effect on the Indian tribes. The idea of sinful behavior suggested by many missionaries made the dividing line between mental illness and social change even more confusing for Indian people.[25] However, toward the end of the

19th century, the religious concepts of illness behavior gave way to a new philosophy of behavior: the idea that biological determinants influenced behavioral patterns. This theory developed as a result of the discovery of the causal link between syphilis and general paresis.[29] Because of this link, many medical people felt that all abnormal behavior would ultimately be linked to some biological disease entity. This perspective was a return to the idea of unity between mind and body, but of a far different type from that practiced by the Indians before contact with Europeans.[35,67,80]

THE ASSIMILATION ERA: 1890–1970

The defeat and total obliteration of the American Indian appeared possible after the Wounded Knee Massacre in 1890.*

* The tragedy of Wounded Knee, 1890, began several years earlier with two significant events, the spreading of the Ghost Dance and the death of the Great Sioux Leader, Sitting Bull. The Ghost Dance was danced to give back strength to the Sioux and to help rid them of the white soldiers. The dance was unfortunately interpreted as a war dance by many whites. Indians, such as Big Foot, who helped spread the practice of the Ghost Dance, were placed on government lists as agitators, and the military was dispatched to Wounded Knee to quell any disturbances. After Sitting Bull was killed, the remaining Sioux were further demoralized, and many, under the leadership of Big Foot (December 1890), started toward Pine Ridge to join with Red Cloud. Along the way, the military intercepted Big Foot's band and ordered them to camp at Wounded Knee. The military leaders had been told to send Big Foot and his people to the military prison, but before this could happen, a tragic misunderstanding occurred.

To ensure that there would be no trouble, Big Foot (who was ill with pneumonia) and his people were ordered to disarm. The soldiers felt that they were not disarming thoroughly enough and began searching the teepees. Angered over the actions of the soldiers, one Indian, Black Coyote, fired his gun. Within minutes, more violence broke out and the soldiers began firing on the Indians with several Hotchkiss guns (Gatling-like guns) that surrounded the Indian encampment. After the shooting ended, at least 300 Sioux men, women and children were dead.[49]

At that time, depression, alcoholism, and violence were found in epidemic proportions on reservations. Although this was not unlike the situation of today, there was a crucial difference. With the eventual settlement of the continent almost accomplished, the plan for the Indian by the federal government changed from one of outright annihilation to the more subtle one of assimilation. The assimilation movement was to last from the late 1800s through the termination movements of the 1960s and 1970s and is still evident in legislation of the present time.[28,34,39]

The concept of assimilation consists of the "mainstreaming" of Indians into white culture and society, something that had been attempted, with mixed success, by the Indian boarding schools.[38] However, assimilation appeared to fail as well. Even with so much of their "Indianness" removed, children were seldom accepted into the white world and were often left in a limbo of what has been called "cultural ambivalence" and/or "cultural discontinuity."[2,52]

The Dawes Act of 1887, also known as the "Allotment Act," gave Indians the right to own and sell their lands on the reservations. The Allotment Act was passed in the hope of encouraging Indians to begin farming with European methods. Unfortunately, what actually happened was increased ownership of Indian lands by non-Indians and further disruption of native life.[40] During the last part of the 19th century, life on reservations was typified by disease and starvation. Indian agents were charged with providing food to the Indians, but more often than not, this did not occur. It seemed that, regardless of the original intent, governmental policy led to the continued death and destruction of native people.[39,53]

The Indians' choices were severe: death or, in order to survive, abandonment of their traditional ways and assimilation into the white culture. Movement away from old traditions was escalated by the deaths of the great chiefs. These chiefs were symbols of the past greatness and cohesion of the tribes, sources of strength and leadership to their people. Each chief's death seemed to signal the further death of all Indians.[38,49]

The psychological state of American Indians during this period has been described as being "helplessly low."[34] Each passing day seemed to have been marked by the government's taking something further from them. The discovery of valuable minerals and energy resources on tribal lands instigated termination of more reservation lands, as happened with the northern half of the Colville Indian reservation in north central Washington. It seemed that no one, including the Indians themselves, cared enough or knew how to stop the downward spiral into oblivion begun years earlier by the epidemics and continued conflict. This trend continued well into the 20th century, until the achievement of U.S. citizenship for Indians in 1924 and the Indian Reorganization Act of 1934.[37,40]

Citizenship and Reorganization: 1924–1934

Full citizenship and voting rights were granted to most tribal members in 1924, the last people to be allowed that privilege in the United States. In 1934 the Indian Reorganization Bill was passed. This bill gave Indians the right to self-government, stipulated a discontinuation of allotments, and established provisions for education and training of American Indians. These two bills assisted reorganization and citizenship and protected the identity of American Indians but failed to end social, health, and governmental problems.

The Great Depression of the 1930s had a long-lasting impact on all people in the United States. Indians living on reservations and practicing subsistence activities may have fared better during these years than much of the rest of the country. Unfortunately, such an advantage was soon destroyed for many Indians with the creation of various federal building projects. The Grand Coulee Dam, for instance, which provided jobs and power in the depressed economy of the Northwest, destroyed the subsistence-based economy of the Indians who resided there. The building of the dam, and the subsequent flooding of 161 square miles of land, inundated farms and orchards, destroyed salmon runs, and drowned the wild plants that provided the earliest source of fresh vegetables in spring.(5) In addition to this tragedy, there was further insult to the native people, who were not included in any of the decision-making processes regarding the building of the dam. It seemed, in spite of the acts of 1924 and 1934, that Indians, their councils, and their means of livelihood were overlooked. For many Indians, particularly those in the Northwest, the loss of the salmon was viewed as a final step toward destruction of their life-style.(25) Early Indian legends spoke of the loss of salmon as the ultimate punishment for misdeeds, and the completion of the Grand Coulee Dam and other dams made this fear a reality.

The early events of World War II speeded the end of the depression and were too pervasive to be ignored. Tribal groups sent their young men to war, and many of them, such as the Navajo talkers, Ira Hayes, and others, became heroes. After World War II, the United States government and the majority of the people once again resumed the notion of the "melting pot," and the American Indian faced one of his most awesome challenges, the era of termination.

Termination and Relocation

After the war, destruction took on a new label in the 1950s with the official federal policy of "termination." Termination consisted of the dissolving of the "special relationship between the Federal government and Indian tribes." The purpose of termination was to bring Indians into the "mainstream" of American life. Concurrent with the termination movement was "relocation," the moving of Indian people previously living on reservation land into the urban centers of the country.[34,37]

The relocation of Indians was intended to assist Indian people by moving them into the cities, where they would find better economic opportunities. Many Indians received training and found jobs through programs established during the social reformation movements of the 1960s. Many more Indians, however, did not successfully make these adjustments and found themselves with no job skills and therefore few economic opportunities. In many instances they could not return to reservation status for economic support. The relocation process may be responsible, in part, for the expanded social welfare problems and increased rates of alcoholism among urban Indians.[54–57]

INDIAN SELF-DETERMINATION

The Indian Self-Determination Act was passed several years after President Nixon's 1970 declaration for greater Indian independence. It was intended to provide Indian people with more control in the development of Federal-Indian programs. Health programs included under this act gave tribes the option of contracting for health services with the Indian Health Service and/or of developing tribal social and health services programs. The Self-Determination Act was followed by the Indian Health Care Improvement Act (1976), which intended to "implement the Federal responsibility for the care and education of the Indian people by improving the services of Federal Indian health programs and encouraging maximum participation of Indians in such programs."[25,27] Both of these acts were designed to include tribal input in the planning and implementation of health, education, and social services programs. These bills, however, were oriented toward administrative responsibilities and did not explicitly address issues such as inclusion of traditional Indian healers in health programs.

These acts have been implemented via the writing of tribal-specific health plans, contracting for services through the Indian Health Service, and setting up tribally supported health programs. The Indian Health Care Improvement Act mandated that tribes write a tribal-specific health plan that would detail the health needs of the community and develop proposals for providing adequate health services. The plans focused upon the leading causes of illness and death for the community, the quality of housing available, and the resources needed to address health issues for the Indian community.[58]

Indian Theories of Mental Health

From 1890 to the present day, the view of mental health and illness has been influenced by Christian dogma, federal government policy, the rapid changes occurring in psychiatry itself, and a complex view of medicine as understood by most Indians. For them, medicine was more than assessment, remedies, and treatment. Medicine was seen as a series of concepts and ideas, and curative medicine was just one form of a broader issue. Religion, magic, spiritism, and divination all play major roles in Indian medicine, and great power was given to the process of healing.[59–63]

The religion and boarding school experiences continued to influence Indian people. The implementation of the Christian philosophy often led to a view of American Indians as inferior, and one might be bad for being Indian and perhaps destined for obliteration.[42] The notion of Indians as inferior and "their mischief and folly" coming from "their barbarous practices" was reinforced by the boarding schools and legislation outlawing Indian languages and religions.[38]

In 1955 the United States Public Health Service assumed responsibility from the Bureau of Indian Affairs for the provision of health care to American Indians, and established the Indian Health Service.[34] The health caregivers were physicians and other professionals trained in the medical model, which produced limited success with Indian people since it neglected many of the social and community influences on native people's lives.[64] The establishment of community health representatives and the inclusion of native healers within the treatment team are efforts on the part of the Indian Health Service to improve care by including the community in the treatment process.

Strong argument can be made for the applicability of psychodynamic concepts to American Indian mental health problems, but this model does not take into account the pervasive influences of Indian society, culture, and environments. One model that does acknowledge these factors is the behavioral view of mental health. The behavioral view and the survival pact of precontact, preepidemic life share many of the same concepts, although superficially they may appear to be quite different. Both models see the cause of behavior as influenced primarily by external events and avoid conceptualization of personality in terms of internal conflicts.[51]

One aspect of the behavioral model is Seligman's[65,66] concept of "learned helplessness." According to Seligman, depression occurs because a person learns he will fail no matter what he attempts. Before contact, rules contained in the survival pact provided the information necessary to sustain life and culture. After contact and imposition of the reservation system, these rules no longer applied, and no matter what was attempted in the next 150 years, most Indians had difficulty in surviving, much less prospering. With this reference, the behavioral model also offers a more appropriate therapeutic approach than does a strict psychoanalytic model. Seligman points out that one way to alleviate depression is to give people success experiences and teach them that they can make valid, viable decisions. The behavioral approach also provides a means for modifying external reinforcers in order to change behavior.

The ecological model of behavior has been previously mentioned as theoretically similar to the survival pact. Both views endorse a symbiotic relationship between the individual and the environment. When symbiosis is disrupted (as from the epidemics, Indian wars, implementation of the reservations, and the termination movements) psychological problems result. The history of the American Indian has been one of constant stresses and change, as described in some tenets of the ecological model—e.g., succession of society.[23] When culture loss was experienced by the tribes, they attempted to fill the void with resources the white society provided, combined with those native traditions left in religion, culture, and government.

The Mental Health Systems Act

Alcoholism, suicide, and violence have been of concern to Indian communities and tribal governments for years, and it was hoped that legislation passed in the 1970s would eventually lead to more effective programs. Meeting the needs of the underserved was a major concern of the Carter administration, and with the underserved in mind, the Mental Health Systems Act of 1980 was passed (PL 96-398). This act provided seed money for start-up of mental health programs for the "chronically underserved," including rural communities and minority groups, a classification that included many American Indians. The Mental Health Act paralleled the Community Mental Health Centers Act of the 1960s in that it advocated the use of community-specific programs and services that were readily accessible to members of that community. The Mental Health Systems Act suggested that "natural helpers" be used in mental health programs but failed to provide the means of incorporating them into future existing programs.

Following the change of the president in 1980, it became evident that the federal administration's fiscal policies would prevent the implementation of the above legislation. The ability of the Indian Health Service to respond to existing health needs, much less develop adequate new programs, was critically eroded by major budget cuts and the apparent lack of interest of federal officials.

TODAY'S MENTAL HEALTH PROBLEMS AND PROGRAMS IN AMERICAN INDIAN COMMUNITIES

Problems

A good deal of attention has been paid to the negative patterns of behavior that Indian people utilized to deal with the stresses in their lives. While alcoholism, violence, and suicide are three of the more destructive coping behaviors, they are also identified as symptoms of some of the critical problems Indian communities face today.[1,3,52,55,67]

The rates of alcoholism, violence, suicide, and accidental death have greatly increased among Indian people in the past 25 years.[1] American Indian people also experienced a higher mortality rate than any other ethnic population group in this country. Many coping methods have remained maladaptive and unproductive; however, these patterns have been so prominent in contemporary Indian life that most Indians experience these behaviors directly or indirectly throughout their lives.

Several theories have been postulated to account for the high rate of destructive behavior in Indian communities. Among them are (a) cultural ambivalence—the psychological state of a person who does not have access to, or identify with, either his own traditional culture or that of the majority culture[2,52]; (b) loss of traditional culture, language, and beliefs; (c) loss of control over one's life (learned helplessness); (d) a learned pattern of passive survival behavior; and (e) a combination of the above-mentioned processes.

Alcoholism

Alcohol abuse remains one of the most pressing problems facing American Indians today. Alcohol use is thought to have first occurred among most Indian tribes with the arrival of early European explorers, traders, and adventurers who used alcohol as barter and as a means for overcoming any "resistance" Indians might have to trade.[15] Subsequent alcohol use and abuse is documented throughout the history of most Indian tribes.[1,62]

Today, alcoholism is cited as being of primary concern among Indian people,[4,54,68] and many differing views of cause and treatment are espoused. One of these views is that alcohol abuse is acquired as a learned pattern of behavior, with role models who teach younger people how and when to drink. If the role models are negative, the learned behavior will also be negative. Bandura's[69] research on modeling has shown that the closer the observer identifies with the modeler, the more likely imitative behavior is to occur. The concept of modeling has great potential for both the treatment and the prevention of alcoholism. If role models can be cultivated who demonstrate positive drinking patterns and positive nondrinking patterns, a more realistic approach to alcohol drinking or abstinence may be established. An effort can be made to outline community-specific rules and standards for drinking and nondrinking behavior.

The prevention and control of alcohol misuse is crucial since increased rates of suicide and violence are found in Indian groups with high rates of alcoholism.[15] Of equal significance remains the control of alcohol abuse among Indian women in order to prevent the fetal alcohol syndrome, a problem that severely limits the physical, social, and intellectual potential of affected children. Finally, alcohol itself accounts for a large number of deaths among Indians and may be viewed as part of the continuing trend of American Indian genocide, initiated by factors that have led to the destruction of the survival pact.[20] Therefore, to improve the physical and mental health of Indian people, new and innovative approaches, using community definitions and personnel, need to be developed for productive treatment of alcohol abuse.

Depression and Low Self-Esteem

Depression is another disorder commonly found in Indian communities. Upon closer examination, it has been found that many Indian people have acquired feelings of inadequacy and low self-worth, often related to experiences in boarding schools that managed to "crush the Indian in each child."[38] Unfortunately, "crushing" the child's spirit also resulted in psychological problems that remain throughout the person's life.[54] The theory of learned helplessness also accounted for a great deal of the depression seen among Indian people.

One means of counteracting depression would be to increase Indian people's success experiences, both on an individual level and as a tribal group. Indian self-determination could lead to group successes. Another approach could be the revision of the curricula of schools by presenting a more positive and accurate picture of Indian Life. Indian and non-Indian children alike need to learn that there *are* many positive aspects to Indian life of which they can be proud.

Perhaps, once the problems of alcoholism, low self-esteem, and depression are adequately addressed, a goodly portion of their destructive results may decrease. There is an enormous need for programs to incorporate the positive aspects of reservation life and Indian culture into existing mental health programs.

Programs now incorporate contemporary Indian elements in an effort to address the problems earlier described. Two of these programs deserve mention: the Navajo School for Medicine Men and the Clinton Indian Hospital in Oklahoma. Both address the issue of integration of culturally relevant elements into their programs but approach the matter from different points of view.

Health Programs and Formal Practices

The Navajo School for Medicine Men began in 1965 as part of the Rough Rock Demonstration School on the Navajo Reservation and received funding from the National Institute of Mental Health (NIMH). Practicing medicine men make up the faculty at the school and determine who will be accepted for training. Training requires a period of several years and consists of learning the diagnostic and treatment methods used by Navajo medicine people. The traditional songs, dances, and medical practices are altered as little as possible to maintain cultural and spiritual integrity.(70,71) Bergman(70,71) presents anecdotal evidence for the success of the school and states that the graduates are well received and frequently used by community members. The funding by NIMH for this program lends credibility for continued use of traditional medicine.

The Clinton Indian Hospital in Clinton, Oklahoma, is another example of the integration of contemporary Indian religious elements into a health care program. A supportive atmosphere using traditional practices aids clients in dealing with day-to-day stress, gives positive feelings about being "Indian," and helps them attain a positive sense of value and direction in their lives.(72)

In another setting, Kemnitzer(73,74) presents a participant observation descriptive analysis of a contemporary Dakota medical system and the cultural milieu within which that system exists, the modern reservation of the northern plains. The study provides a background on contemporary Dakota culture, technical aspects of the Yuwipi during ritual, theoretical concepts that guide the form of the rituals, and documentation of the social position of the practitioners in society. Elements such as these are important in planning for local health services.

Finally, the Native American Church has been viewed positively as dealing with the problem of alcoholism among Indians, although criticized because of the use of peyote.* Albaugh and Anderson(72) point out that this is not the only factor in alcoholism treatment. Rather, they indicate that it is the format of the NAC that allows for open expression of feelings and a decrease in people's sense of alienation, which in turn encourages development of more positive coping mechanisms and self-concepts. Albaugh and Anderson believe that the inclusion of cultural elements, such as the tenets of the NAC, provide an important resource in treating alco-

* The actual use of peyote in this program is limited and done under the strict guidelines of the NAC.

holism in American Indians. Time will determine the value of these programmatic efforts, and, if successful, the concept can be used in a variety of programs in different Indian communities.

Amoss[47,48] points out that Spirit Dancing is an effort at resurrecting the concept of kinship that was so important to Indians in precontact, preepidemic tribal life.[10,16] Through dancing, efforts are made at resolving conflicting cultural issues—e.g., individual autonomy as espoused in Western culture, as opposed to kin solidarity important in traditional Indian culture. Resolution is accomplished by having one's own song, dance, and spirit, and by using one's family and kin for support and help during the dance. The symbiotic relationship between the individual and the group affirms the intricate but necessary relationship among all group members. The economic functions of Spirit Dancing have changed over the past 100 years as tribal survival shifted from subsistence to commodity and cash economies. Food, blankets, and other necessities for dancing are provided by members of the community, who donate whatever surpluses are available. Such cooperation helps to reinforce the ties within the group and provides resources for payment to special orators, as well as being an aid to less fortunate members of the community. The Spirit Dance has a social function that strengthens group ties in a fashion similar to that of the traditional economic and kin solidarity functions. The positive social function of the dance is exemplified in its having solidified the numerous small coastal Salish Indian groups in the Northwest. It also provides young people an opportunity to meet prospective marriage partners.[47,48] The potency of Spirit Dancing as a means of group cohesion and individual expression is part of what makes it an attractive practice. Four key components of Spirit Dancing can be identified that may have some implications for existing and future mental health and social programs in Indian communities. These components are (a) focus on individual autonomy, (b) strong kinship ties, (c) community unification and affirmation of ancestral continuity, and (d) guidelines and options for behaviors. These components are very important when discussing treatment options for chronic behavioral disturbances in any culture.

"TRADITIONAL" DEFINITIONS OF SICKNESS AND TYPES OF HEALING

The four-author study on Piman shamanism and staying sickness (Ka:cim Mumkidag)[75,76] is a landmark in the investigation of the basic concepts of one American Indian tribe's theory of human health and illness.[43,69] The study describes a healing tradition, little affected by other cultural forces. The study is based on a series of sessions in which questions are asked by three of the authors, with answers provided by the fourth, Juan Gregorio, a practicing Papago Makai (shaman). The theory and concepts underlying the actual processes of curing the Pima's culturally bound illness category of Ka:cim Mumkidag (staying sickness) is addressed. Ka:cim Mumkidag is the result of violations of the code of life set down in the beginning by the Piman creator, I:toi. All other categories of sickness can afflict any human, Piman and non-Piman. Another example in the same tradition is a Northern Cheyenne ethnopsychology study that focuses on concepts of self and person to explain individual social behavior in terms of Cheyenne cultural theory. The basic concept of good physical health is tied to spiritual well-being.[21]

Comparative studies of native and Euro-American mental health practices are also reported in the scientific literature.[30,60–63,77,78] There is a basic problem in comparative studies that is difficult to overcome: A simple one-to-one or direct relationship between the diagnostic categories of two cultures does not exist. Each system arises from different views of reality, different theories of physiology, and different etiologies. The two systems of thought, however, are not necessarily in conflict, since both are applicable simultaneously, but separately, to the same illness phenomena. For example, Jilek[60–63] found indications that the Guardian Spirit Ceremonies are effective for two symptom complexes: psychoneurotic and psychophysiologic syndromes, and antisocial, aggressive behavior, frequently associated with drug or alcohol abuse. According to Jilek,[60–63] both syndromes were found to be frequently related to anomic depression.

Acosta[79] describes an interesting perspective by workers on the Southwestern Zuni Pueblo approach to community mental health. A complex network of permanent treatment groups meets both the moral exigencies of the belief system and the requirements of social order in the Zuni tribe. The groups are made up of lifelong members who are devoted to the management of chronic behavior disorders. The concept of community mental health fits Zuni social organization. Under the traditional Zuni system, deviant behavior has been systematically incorporated into the ongoing daily social arrangements of Zuni society. Incorporation of such behavior is accomplished without show of force or hardship to individuals in Clown Fraternities. The Clown Fraternities are a complex of groups whose activities are legitimized by ancient Zuni myth and ritual. The supernatural figures associated with the fraternities provide behavioral models for the characters of the sacred dance dramas, as well as for the recruitment of likely members. The purpose of the associations is not to stop the problem behavior but rather to control it in such a way that it can be placed in its proper niche as seen by the community. Individuals who join the fraternities may continue to exhibit problem behavior, but under the aegis of the fraternity, such behavior is controlled and turned to the good of the community in public performances and secret rituals. Thus, individuals classified as severely retarded, alcoholic, or epileptic find a useful role within the complex organization of Zuni society.

Camazine's[80] review of the practices of the individual healers of Zuni medicine societies explores the use of two alternative health care systems by the people of Zuni Pueblo. These practitioners treat sorcery, disease object intrusion, and breach of taboo cases. Health problems not considered to be of supernatural origin are traditionally treated by folk remedies. Camazine views the Zuni situation as one in which scientific medicine is replacing the medicine societies and which is now in a transitional period. The traditional Zuni medical system is seen by practitioners of Western medicine as benign, with some placebo effects, and is therefore considered complementary to scientific medicine.

Neutra, Levy, and Parker[67] followed 10 patients for 11 years who were diagnosed as epileptics or as having hysterical seizures. Interestingly, these patients' symptoms resembled three seizure syndromes recognized by the Navajos: I chaa (generalized seizures with incest as the cause and accompanied by considerable social stigma); frenzy witchcraft (characterized by fugue states and caused by witchcraft); and hand trembling (considered to be a sign of shamanistic tendencies). The investigators tested medically diagnosed persons against the cultural epileptic syndrome of the Navajo and found that the frequency and pattern of epilepsy and hysteria among Navajo are noticeably different from those in other populations. Diagnosed hysterics did show some tendency toward attempting the role of the hand trembler. None, however, remained in the role, which would appear to indicate that despite external signs of shamanistic potential, overt hysterics are not suitable candidates for this role.

Wagner[81] reports that Navajos use curing services from scientific medicine, the Peyote religion, fundamentalist Christianity, and traditional Navajo medicine interchangeably. Decisions as to which source of healing is to be used are situational and based on financial costs, length of treatment time, probable effectiveness, and accessibility of services.

BENEFITS OF INTEGRATION

There are practical benefits of integration and incorporation of all available mental-health-related functions into one community system of mutually understood responsibilities and capabilities with cross-referral opportunities and positively sanctioned status for all. The development of such a comprehensive mental health system could provide services appropriate to all segments of the community. A major problem identified by mental health professionals remains the cultural differences between professionals and patient.(83) Lack of the cultural perspective in diagnosis, with potential negative treatment prescriptions, is well documented in the mental health literature.(60,84) Lewis(83) has written of his experience, as a practicing psychiatrist, with an ailment prevalent in the Lakota tribe, the Wacinko syndrome (very similar to reactive depression and the soul-loss syndrome, with loss of appetite and sleep, sometimes leading to suicide). Lewis found that Lakota practitioners are more successful in treatment of Wacinko than is conventional drug-based mental health therapy. It would seem very practical for a mental health service unit to be able to use this type of culture-specific information in referral and treatment.

The usefulness of cultural information in terms of patient care begins with the intake process and continues through diagnosis. Shore(84) has recommended that "diagnosis can be strengthened by the participation of mental health workers experienced with American Indians (professionals, paraprofessionals, and people involved in traditional medicine) in the evaluative process to provide a cultural perspective for the psychiatric diagnostician."

What is the status of American Indian medicine in contemporary communities? Is traditional medicine an anachronistic cultural remnant, or is there still something to be identified as Indian medicine? Viable contemporary folk medicine in American Indian communities exists that is a synthesis of many components, including traditional Indian medicine. Many Indian health caregivers support Jilek's[60–63] argument that there is a renaissance of American Indian therapeutic self-help. In summarizing, he states: "The persistence and revival of indigenous American Indian healing is due, not to lack of modern treatment services, but to a need for culture-cogenial and holistic therapeutic approaches, such as those conceptualized by transcultural psychiatry and psychosomatic medicine but still rarely applied in practice."

The 1981 National Indian Health Conference included a panel discussion of the role of traditional Indian medicine in contemporary health services delivery. The panelists seem to have generally advocated the incorporation of traditional Indian medicine practices into an integrated system with scientific medicine. They also indicated that integration has not yet taken place for at least two reasons: skepticism on the part of scientific medical practitioners, and a lack of information about traditional medicine by many Indians. A third obstacle, not as clearly stated, is a reluctance of at least some traditional practitioners to become involved with Euro-American medicine, as is suggested in an ongoing survey by Willard and LaDue.[29] The survey offers some preliminary indications of the extent of integration of the two systems. Urban programs are reported as being involved in networks of referrals and services of a great variety, but no native medicine involvement has yet been mentioned. Reservation-oriented and

-based programs report working with Indian medicine practitioners in informal relationships, with positive community sanctions for that involvement. A small number indicate formal involvement of native medicine practitioners.

METHODS OF INTEGRATION

The options for incorporation of native medicine practitioners into mental health services systems include (1) integration of native practitioners directly into system services, (2) incorporation of practitioners as determined by professional and community board certification, (3) continuation of the present informal referral system, and (4) development and acceptance of traditional healers by the health care establishment, and encouragement of referrals.

The community's integration of native medicine into mental health services is a most important process that will provide sanction and support for programs and help identify legitimate healers. Evidence points to an increased use of traditional healers among both urban and reservation Indians. Urban Indians who return to reservations desire access to both traditional and Western healing.[38] Community support and sanction are also derived through resolutions passed by tribal councils and local Indian health boards.[85] This support by the community is essential if integration of traditional medicine is to occur.

It is crucial that people in the community are able to have an input into any programs being designed for them. A community needs assessment involving Indian residents of the community, and a community board of directors for mental health services would be a good start. Such involvement could personalize health programs for their community. Significantly, it would allow participants to identify strengths and positive aspects about themselves and their community that could be incorporated into the treatment program. The incorporation of native medicine practitioners into mental health services of the Indian Health Service will require policy alterations and funding support at the director's level. Mental health departments will need clear mandates as to the types of services provided to the community. Staff must be flexible enough to welcome the inclusion of traditional and natural helpers as viable and useful components of the treatment team. Other issues involved in integration at the agency level are training, referral, and personnel selection. Both selection and acceptance of healers may offer problems to trained Western agency personnel. With loss of the traditional development of healers and/or shamans, it has become necessary to provide training for this role. The Navajo School for Medicine Men(71) is one of the few institutions that offers training on a *formal* basis.

It is the contention of many health caregivers that the capabilities of existing mental health services for American Indians are increasingly overtaxed. Indications that there will be no improvement of these services in the immediate future are abundant. Exploration of potential extension of mental health services by linkages to existing community resources, through involvement of both traditional and nontraditional healers, and evaluations of existing community support groups are now occurring. Integration will tap the enormous strengths that exist in Indian communities, strengths that may be missed by conventional practitioners. The ultimate goal of all social and health programs is to produce a healthy people, and integration of traditional healing services is one avenue to develop strong people and provide necessary treatment.

Other Therapeutic Techniques

The incorporation of traditional healing as a part of comprehensive mental health does not obviate the use of familiar therapeutic techniques generally used with disadvantaged families. Often a concrete, problem-solving approach that provides patients with workable solutions to their problems is the approach of choice. Problem-solving therapy seems to be particularly useful in sorting out multiproblems in family counseling. Many families seek help when their present methods of coping collapse and a crisis occurs.

A family crisis may be precipitated by an event influenced by several underlying issues. It is a challenge for the therapist to identify the precipitating event and to explore its significance with the family. Such exploration may consume several hours in which the therapist acts as clarifier, validator, negotiator, and educator. Adequate time and flexibility are crucial if the therapist is to help the family obtain a clear understanding of their problem and develop alternate coping mechanisms.

In individual therapy, concrete, problem-solving therapy can be used on both a long- and short-term basis. In the initial session the therapist may assume an active role as problem identifier, reality tester, facilitator, limit setter. While such an approach may be more directive than that of many therapists, it does assist the patient in externalizing conflicts more easily. In other instances, nondirective therapy based on Maslow's hierarchy of needs is useful in outlining basic survival issues and needs for Indian people, a large number of whom are still far below the poverty level. The consequences of unmet needs could be marital discord, violence, and/or heavy drinking, which result from the need for a release of some of the stresses of poverty. The therapist, in this situation, may become an educator—i.e., explaining the necessity of having one's basic needs met, and how, if they are not met, large amounts of tension, poor self-concept, and other negative methods of coping can develop. When the client has a grasp of how tension results from unmet needs, progression to a problem-solving, limit-setting, or traditional Indian methods of therapy can follow. The therapist may also be a liaison for the client, helping him or her to obtain employment or needed social services. Flexibility of the therapist and knowledge of the community is extremely important since many Indian people may be reluctant to seek out help due to past negative experiences with governmental bureaucracies. A desire to solve problems without outside help may also keep Indians from making use of available facilities.

All therapy approaches, regardless of the underlying theory, offer the patient a means of understanding his or her needs and pressures. Development of positive coping mechanisms is more likely once understanding occurs. The therapist must be willing to use a variety of techniques and resources to aid the client and must be prepared to meet with clients in many settings—e.g., hospitals, jails, taverns, or the client's home.

FUTURE DIRECTIONS

The emphasis on future mental health programs should be based on community concepts of problems *and* strengths. More research is needed to determine these issues and to help design community-specific programs. Health care professionals and academicians need to be willing to use and incorporate community knowledge and develop natural helping systems in these communities. The uniqueness of the culture of the American Indian needs to be understood, and *all* research projects require cooperation with both tribal government and community people. Research on community-derived problems can then be given to tribal systems to use in future program design and implementation. For example, many tribes possess vast natural resources, and as these are developed, the impact of industrialization and sudden wealth on the people of the area will require continuous monitoring as a step to prevent problems.

As a corollary, *no* federal legislation should be enacted, whether in energy, economic, or human resources development, without the intimate involvement of the Indian people it will affect. For too long, the federal government has done just this with disastrous results. Indian people can and should make the decisions that will lead to greater self-esteem and improved health. Indian self-determination, after 200 years, must become a reality, and mental health professionals can be important in their work with and for Indian people.

APPENDIX

Chronology(25,31,36,37,38)

1519 Public burning of Indian Chiefs by Cortés.

1622 Powhatan's feeding of Virginia settlers.

1763 Treaty which closed western areas to white settlement.

1775 Continental Congress assumes control of Indian affairs and names commissioners for the northern, middle, and southern departments.

1786–1789 A series of treaties establishes a policy of acquiring Indian lands by purchase rather than by right of conquest.

1797 Northwest Ordinance of July 13, 1797: "The utmost good faith shall always be observed towards the Indians . . . ," etc.

1789 Under the Constitution, Article I, Section 8, Clause 3, the Congress is given the specific authority to "regulate commerce with foreign nations, and among the several States, and with the Indian tribes."

1789 Under the Constitution, the Congress continues the use of the secretary of war to manage Indian affairs.

1789 In four statutes the Congress establishes federal authority to make war (or presumably peace), to govern territories, to make treaties, and to spend money in dealing with Indians.

1790 End of first smallpox epidemic, begun in 1782—loss of 80% and more of tribal populations in the Pacific Northwest.

1792 Exploration and mapping of the northwest coast by George Vancouver lead to more settling and opening of lands to fur traders in the future.

1803 As a result of the Louisiana Purchase from France, a vast new territory with a large Indian population is added to the United States, and Thomas Jefferson proposes the removal of eastern Indians to the area west of the Mississippi.

1803–1806 The Lewis and Clark Expedition contacts many new Indian tribes as it explores the region from the Mississippi River to the Pacific Ocean for the United States.

1811 Building of Fort Astoria by Astor Fur Company.

1812–1825 Gradual withdrawal of European claims in the Northwest, ending the period of relatively peaceful trade in the area and beginning the push to fulfill America's "Manifest Destiny" to stretch across the continent.

1824 The Secretary of War creates a Bureau of Indian Affairs within the War Department.

1829–1831 Second wave of epidemics, of "intermittent fever," further decimation of the Pacific Northwest tribes, again by as much as 80%, opening up more lands and giving more space for the increasing occupation by whites.

1830 Indian Removal Act passed by the Congress (Trail of tears).

1832 Office of Commissioner of Indian Affairs created within the War Department.

1834 Indian Trade and Intercourse Act redefines Indian country and introduces significant changes through reorganization of the Indian Service.

1837 Simultaneous building of the Whitman mission in the interior and the Blanchet and Demers mission on the coast begins the long-reaching influence of the Protestant and Catholic religions—also start of seeing a decline of the Northwest tribes as "preordained" and inevitable, with the responsibility of helping the tribes go into oblivion as peacefully as possible.

1849 Homestead Act—opening up land for settlement, ignoring the Indians' claims of territory, hunting, and fishing rights.

1851 Dart treaties, which tried to stave off some of the mistakes of the federal and territorial governments; none of these ratified, and removal of tribes continues.

1853 Washington Territory is created.

1864 Massacre at Sand Creek

1867–1868 Indian Peace Commission negotiates final treaties with Indians (last of 370 with the Nez Perce on August 13, 1868).

1869 President Grant's so-called Peace policy inaugurated.

1869 Act creating Board of Indian Commissioners (continued until eliminated by executive order in 1933).

1870–1876 Following federal Indian policy, the remaining tribes are placed on reservations, with the help of the military when necessary. Rations of food and clothing are made available in lieu of the privilege of hunting in "customary places."

1870s Beginnings of a federal program to provide schools for the education of Indians.

1871 The negotiation of treaties between the United States and Indian tribes is ended by congressional action.

1877 Nez Perce War, flight of Chief Joseph.

1878 Congress authorizes the establishment of a United States Indian Police.

1883 Courts of Indian Offenses are authorized to allow tribal units to administer justice in all but the major crimes.

1885 United States courts are given jurisdiction over Indian cases involving major crimes (murder, manslaughter, rape, assault with intent to kill, arson, burglary, and larceny).

1887 The General Allotment or Dawes Severalty Act makes the allotment of land to individual Indians and the breaking up of tribal landholdings the official policy of the United States.

1889 Two million acres of Oklahoma Territory are bought from the Indians and opened for settlement.

1890 Wounded Knee Massacre.

1891 Provision is made for the leasing of allotted Indian lands.

1902–1910 Beginnings of federal Indian reclamation, forestry, and conservation programs.

1904 Death of Chief Joseph.

1906 The Burke Act amends certain features of the Dawes Act on allotment, and defines Indian "competency."

1907 The Supreme Court defines the right of the United States to reserve waters for the use of Indian tribes in *Winters v. United States* (so-called Winters Doctrine).

1909–1912 Beginnings of a formal Indian health program, with a special message from President Taft to the Congress on that subject August 10, 1912.

1924 The Congress grants citizenship to Indians. A majority were already citizens as a result of treaties or earlier blanket grants to particular groups. (Indians did not gain the right to vote in all states, however, until 1948.)

1924 A Division of Indian Health is established within the Bureau of Indian Affairs.

1928 The Meriam Report on the *Problem of Indian Administration* is published, after a 2-year study, recommending various reforms and changes of policy in Indian affairs.

1928–1943 The Senate Committee on Indian Affairs conducts a survey of Indian programs and policies that has far-reaching repercussions.

1931 $50,000 is appropriated to secure remunerative employment through the Bureau of Indian Affairs' new Guidance and Placement Division.

1931 A new Division of Agriculture Extension and Industries is established within the Bureau of Indian Affairs.

1932 Leavitt Act frees the Indians from liens on allotted lands totaling millions of dollars. The *Preston–Engle Report* had recommended such action along with a complete reorganization of Indian irrigation services and the abandonment of useless projects.

1933 Steps are taken to emphasize the right of Indians to practice their own customs and religion and to stress the fact that interference with such practices will no longer be tolerated.

1934 New Indian legislation such as the Wheeler-Howard or Indian Reorganization Act officially reverses the trend to break up tribal governments and landholdings typical of the allotment period (1887–1933), provides for tribal self-government, and launches an Indian credit program.

1934 Start of Grand Coulee Dam.

1935 An act to establish an Indian Arts and Crafts Board (accomplished in 1936).

1937 The Bureau of Indian Affairs reports that total Indian landholdings have increased 2,100,000 acres since 1935.

1943–1944 The Bureau of Indian Affairs calls for the preparation of basic development programs by each tribe, band, or group to "facilitate the Federal Government in dispatching its obligations to the Indian. . . ."

1944 The National Congress of American Indians is organized at Denver, Colorado.

1944–1947 The House Indian Affairs Committee conducts its own investigations of government Indian policies.

1945 By the close of World War II it is apparent that experience gained by thousands of Indians on the work relief programs of the 1930s, and by some 65,000 who left reservations to join the armed services or for war work in cities, has wrought considerable change that will strongly affect future Indian actions throughout the United States.

1946 Act to create an Indian Claims Commission to hear claims of Indian tribes against the United States.

1947 The Senate Committee on the Post Office and Civil Service calls for testimony from the Bureau of Indian Affairs on the readiness of particular tribes to have the services of the Indian Bureau withdrawn.

1948 The Hoover Commission recommends the transfer of the Bureau of Indian Affairs to the Federal Security Agency and states that "assimilation must be the dominant goal of public policy" for Indians.

1948–1953 The Bureau of Indian Affairs' job placement program evolves into the "Relocation" program for Indians.

1948–1959 By legislation and administrative action, policy on sale and leasing of individually held Indian land, and on using such land as security for loans, is liberalized from the 1933 to 1945 position.

1949 Representatives of the Bureau of Indian Affairs ask Indian tribes to assist with the development of programs that will help the Indian Bureau "to work itself out of a job."

1949–1964 Rehabilitation payments of over $60 million made to seven tribes displaced in various ways by federal irrigation projects constructed on Indian reservations that were largely beneficial to non-Indians.

1951 The Bureau of Indian Affairs states as program objectives "a standard of living for Indians comparable with that enjoyed by other elements of our society," and the "step-by-step transfer of Bureau functions to the Indians themselves or to appropriate agencies of local, State or Federal Government."

1952 A Division of Programs is established by the Bureau of Indian Affairs to work with individual tribes to achieve the goals stated in 1951 (above).

1953 Congressional action changes discriminatory liquor laws as they pertain to Indians.

1954 Act to transfer the Division of Indian Health from the Bureau of Indian Affairs to the U.S. Public Health Service (PHS) (accomplished in 1955). Appropriations for Indian Health rise from over $12 million in 1950 to over $61 million in 1965.

1954 Legislation to secure transfer of Bureau of Indian Affairs agricultural extension to the Department of Agriculture fails enactment but is later accomplished by administrative action.

1956 The Bureau of Indian Affairs initiates a program to provide basic education to adult Indians, the Congress enacts a vocational training program for Indians from 18 to 35, and the Bureau of Indian Affairs commences an industrial development program to encourage industry to locate on or near Indian reservations and to employ Indian labor.

1957 Legislation authorizes PHS to assist communities with the construction of health facilities that would benefit both Indians and non-Indians.

1958 Legislation allows Indian tribes to benefit from federally impacted area bills (PL 81-815 and PL 81-874) by securing financial assistance for the construction and operation of schools that would benefit Indians.

1958 A statement of the secretary of the interior modifies the position of the department on termination.

1959 Legislation authorizes PHS to construct sanitary facilities for Indians.

1961 Interior Department and Bureau of Indian Affairs change their land sales policy to allow Indian tribes or other Indians the first opportunity to acquire individually owned lands offered for sale by Indians—this is a great assistance in tribal land-consolidation programs.

1961 Interior secretary names a task force to study Indian affairs and make long-range recommendations; the Commission on the Rights, Liberties, and Responsibilities of the American Indian publish their *Program for Indian Citizens;* and Indians gather at Chicago to make their *Declaration of Indian Purpose.*

1964 The Economic Opportunity Act through the Office of Economic Opportunity (OEO), Indian Desk, extends its benefits to Indian reservations.

1966 The appointment of a new commissioner brings a flurry of congressional interest in termination that eventually results in further stress on Indian economic development.

1966 Special programs for Indian children are provided under the Elementary and Secondary Education Act.

1968 Civil Rights Act extends the guarantee of certain constitutional rights to Indians under tribal governments, repeals 1953 action allowing states to extend legal jurisdiction over Indian reservations without tribal consent.

1968 Special message to the Congress on "The Forgotten American" March 6, 1968, by President Lyndon B. Johnson, in which he calls for the establishment of a National Council on Indian Opportunity to be chaired by the vice-president and to include "a cross section of Indian leaders" and the secretaries or directors of those departments or agencies that are significantly involved with Indian programs (NCIO is to encourage all government agencies to make their services available to Indians, and is to coordinate their efforts to achieve particular purposes). President Johnson also suggests that the idea of "termination" should be replaced by Indian "self-determination."

1968 As a presidential candidate, Richard M. Nixon also speaks out against the termination philosophy and suggests that "American society can allow many different cultures to flourish in harmony."

1969 Ninth Circuit Court upholds land "freeze" order of the interior secretary on behalf of native Alaskans and affirms the validity of the native's position in regard to aboriginal use and occupancy.

1969 Environmental Policy Act protects resources of native Americans and other citizens.

1969–1970 Studies of and hearings on urban Indian programs tend to liberalize government services to this group.

1969–1970 It has become Bureau of Indian Affairs policy to encourage the formation of Indian school boards and to invite Indian leaders to take over the management of their own schools and other programs formerly administered by Bureau of Indian Affairs employees.

1970 New census records approximately a 50% increase in the population of native Americans from 1960 to 1970 (1960 count 551,669, compared to a 1970 count of 827,901).

1970 In a special message to Congress on Indian Affairs July 8, 1970, President Nixon states: "The time has come to break decisively with the past and to create conditions for a new era in which the Indian future is determined by Indian acts and Indian decisions." The president also asks for a new concurrent resolution that would "renounce, repudiate, and repeal" the termination policy outlined in HCR 108 of the 83rd Congress.

1970–1971 There is a considerable increase in the number of Indians in leadership positions in federal Indian programs.

1974 Boldt Fishing Rights Decision.

1975 Indian Self-Determination Act.

1976 Indian Health Care Improvement Act of 1975.

1978 Indian Child Welfare Act.

1978 Indian Religious Freedom Act.

REFERENCES

1. C. J. Frederick, *Suicide, Homicide and Alcoholism among American Indians: Guidelines for Help*, National Institute of Mental Health, Rockville, Maryland, 1973.
2. L. French, Social problems among Cherokee females: A study of cultural ambivalence and role identity, *American Journal of Psychoanalysis* 36:163–169, 1976.
3. Indian Health Service Task Force on Alcoholism, *Alcoholism: A High Priority Health Problem*, U.S. Department of Health, Education and Welfare, Washington, D.C., 1977.
4. J. Leland, *Firewater Myths*, Rutgers Center of Alcohol Studies, New Brunswick, New Jersey, 1976.
5. A. Anastasio, *The Southern Plateau: An Ecological Analysis of Intergroup Relations*, University of Idaho, Moscow, Idaho, 1972.
6. C. L. Attneave, Medicine men and psychiatrists in the Indian Health Service, *Psychiatric Annals* 4:49–55, 1974.
7. J. F. Bryde, *Modern Indian Psychology*, Institute of Indian Studies, University of South Dakota, Vermillion, 1971.
8. B. Steiger, *Medicine Talk*, Doubleday, New York, 1975.
9. M. Zax and E. L. Cowen, *Abnormal Psychology: Changing Conceptions*, Holt, Rinehart and Winston, New York, 1972.
10. C. B. Bagley, *Indian Myths of the Northwest*, Lowman & Hanford, Seattle, 1972.
11. J. Bierhorst (ed.), *The Red Swan*, Farrar, Straus & Giroux, New York, 1976.
12. W. H. Capps (ed.), *Seeing with a Native Eye*, Harper & Row, New York, 1976.

13. A. Carmichael, *Indian Legends of Vancouver Island,* Musson, Toronto, 1922.
14. P. Drucker, *Cultures of the North Pacific Coast,* Chandler, San Francisco, 1965.
15. G. W. Fuller, *A History of the Pacific Northwest,* Knopf, New York, 1931.
16. E. Gunther, *Indian Life on the Northwest Coast of North America,* University of Chicago Press, Chicago, 1972.
17. P. Liberty, Priest and shaman on the plains: A false dichotomy, *Plains Anthropologist* 15:73–79, 1970.
18. K. B. Judson, *Myths and Legends of the Pacific Northwest,* A. C. McClurg, Chicago, 1910.
19. W. S. Phillips, *Totem Tales,* Star, Chicago, 1896.
20. V. Deloria, *Behind the Trail of Broken Treaties,* Delacorte Press, New York, 1974.
21. A. S. Strauss, Northern Cheyenne ethnopsychology, *Ethos* 9:326–357, 1977.
22. S. Thompson, *Motif-Index of Folk Literature,* University of Indiana Press, Bloomington, 1955.
23. P. A. Mann, *Community Psychology: Concepts and Applications,* Free Press, New York, 1978.
24. B. L. Bloom, *Community Mental Health: A General Introduction,* Brooks/Cole, Monterey, California, 1977.
25. V. Deloria, *Indians of the Pacific Northwest,* Doubleday, New York, 1977.
26. B. J. Stern, *The Lumni Indians of Northwest Washington,* AMS Press, New York, 1934.
27. W. T. Corlett, *The Medicine Man of the American and His Cultural Background,* Charles C Thomas, Springfield, Illinois, 1935.
28. V. J. Vogel, *American Indian Medicine,* University of Oklahoma Press, Norman, 1970.
29. W. Willard and R. A. LaDue, *Coyote returns: An integration of "old" and "new" medicine in American Indian mental health* (Part 3), Presented at the American Political Science Association Indian Policy Network, New York, September 1981.
30. H. Fabrega and D. G. Silver, *Illness and Shamanistic Curing in Zinacantan: An Ethno Medical Analysis,* Stanford University Press, Stanford, 1973.
31. V. Deloria, *Custer Died for Your Sins,* Avon Books, New York, 1969.
32. H. C. Taylor and L. L. Hoaglen, The "intermittent fever" epidemic of the 1830's on the lower Columbia River, in: *Rolls of Certain Indian Tribes in Washington and Oregon* (C. E. McSheney, ed.), Ye Galleon Press, Fairfield, Washington, 1969.
33. J. Lawson, *History of North Carolina, 1714,* Reprinted by Richmond, Garrett and Massie, Durham, 1937.
34. M. S. Garbarino, *Native American Heritage,* Little, Brown, Boston, 1976.

35. R. H. Glassey, *Pacific Northwest Indian Wars*, Binfods & Mott, Portland, 1953.
36. C. E. McSheney, *Rolls of Certain Indian Tribes in Washington and Oregon*, Ye Galleon Press, Fairfield, Washington, 1969.
37. S. L. Tykler, *A History of Indian Policy*, U.S. Department of the Interior, Washington, D.C., 1973.
38. M. Gidley, *With One Sky Above Us*, Putnam's, New York, 1979.
39. A. L. Getty and D. B. Smith, *One Century Later*, University of British Columbia Press, Vancouver, 1977.
40. K. R. Philip, *John Collier's Crusade for Indian Reform*, University of Arizona Press, Tucson, 1977.
41. A. C. Harrison and J. Marcelley, *Self-Concept as Perceived by Fifteen Native Americans*, Unpublished paper, 1977.
42. S. A. Hayes, *The Resistance to Education for Assimilation by the Colville Indians, 1872–1972*, Spokane School District 81, Spokane, 1972.
43. M. D. Beal, *I Will Fight No More Forever*, Ballantine Books, New York, 1963.
44. M. H. Brown, *The Flight of the Nez Perce*, Putnam's, New York, 1967.
45. W. LaBarre, *The Ghost Dance*, Delta Books, New York, 1970.
46. W. LaBarre, *The Peyote Cult*, Anchor Books, Hamden, Connecticut, 1975.
47. P. T. Amoss, Strategies of orientation: The contribution of contemporary winter dancing to coast Salish identity and solidarity, *Artic Anthropologist* 14:77–83, 1977.
48. P. T. Amoss, *Coast Salish Spirit Dancing: The Survival of an Ancestral Religion*, University of Washington Press, Seattle, 1978.
49. D. Brown, *Bury My Heart at Wounded Knee*, Bantam Books, New York, 1971.
50. L. Lamphere, Symbolic elements in Navajo ritual, *Southwest Journal of Anthropology* 25:279–305, 1969.
51. W. S. Sahakian, *Psychopathology Today: Experimentation and Research*, F. E. Peacock, Itasca, Illinois, 1970.
52. A. Metcalf, From schoolgirl to mother: The effect of education on Navajo women, *Social Problems* 23:533–544, 1976.
53. J. B. Neihardt, *Black Elk Speaks*, University of Nebraska Press, Lincoln, 1961.
54. R. C. Covington, *Red Cloud Was Right: A Position Paper on Colville Mental Health Status and Needs*, Colville Confederated Tribes, Nespelem, Washington, 1977.
55. First Convocation of American Indian Scholars, *Indian Voices*, Indian Historian Press, San Francisco, 1970.
56. N. O. Lurie, The world's oldest on-going protest demonstration: North American Indian drinking patterns, in: *The American Indian* (N. Hundley, ed.), CLIO Books, Santa Barbara, 1974.

57. E. H. Spicer (ed.), *Perspective in American Indian Culture Change*, University of Chicago Press, Chicago, 1961.
58. Colville Confederated Tribes, *Colville Confederate Tribal Health Plan*, Nespelem, Washington, 1979.
59. D. P. Jewell, A case of a psychotic Navajo male, *Human Organization.* 11:32–36, 1952.
60. L. Jilek, The Western psychiatrist and his non-Western clientel: Transcultural experience of relevance to psychotherapy with Canadian Indian patients, *Canadian Psychiatric Association Journal* 21:353–354, 1976.
61. W. G. Jilek, *Salish Indian Mental Health and Culture Change: Psychogenic and Therapeutic Aspects of the Guardian Spirit Ceremonial*, Holt, Rinehart & Winston, Toronto, 1974.
62. W. G. Jilek, Indian healing power: Indigenous therapeutic practices in the Pacific Northwest, *Psychiatric Annals* 4:13–21, 1974.
63. W. G. Jilek and N. Todd, Witchdoctors succeed where doctors fail: Psychotherapy among coast Salish Indians, *Canadian Psychiatric Association Journal* 19:351–356, 1974.
64. M. Beiser and E. Degroat, Body and spirit medicine: Conversations with a Navajo singer, *Psychiatric Annals* 4:9–12, 1974.
65. W. R. Miller and M. E. P. Seligman, Depression and learned helplessness in man, *Journal of Abnormal Psychology* 84:228–238, 1975.
66. W. R. Miller and M. E. P. Seligman, Learned helplessness, depression and the perception of reinforcement, *Behaviour Research and Therapy* 14:7–17, 1976.
67. R. Neutra, J. E. Levy, and D. Parker, Cultural expectations versus reality: Navajo seizure patterns and sick roles, *Culture, Medicine and Psychiatry* 1:255–275, 1977.
68. E. G. Peniston and T. R. Burns, An alcoholic dependency behavior inventory for native Americans, *White Cloud Journal* 1:11–15, 1980.
69. A. Bandura, Behavior theory and the models of man, *American Psychologist* 29:859–869, 1974.
70. R. L. Bergman, Navajo medicine and psychoanalysis, *Human Behavior* 2:8–15, 1973.
71. R. L. Bergman, A school for medicine men, *American Journal of Psychiatry* 130:663–666, 1973.
72. B. J. Albaugh and P. Anderson, Peyote in the treatment of alcoholism among American Indians, *American Journal of Psychiatry* 131:1247–1250, 1974.
73. L. S. Kemnitzer, *Sioux medical care systems*, Paper presented at the Society for Applied Anthropology Annual Meeting, 1971.
74. L. S. Komnitzer, Structure, content, and cultural meaning of Yuwipi: A modern Lakota healing ritual, *American Ethnologist* 3:261–279, 1976.
75. D. M. Bahr, J. Gregori, D. I. Lopez, and A. Alvarez, *Piman Shamanism and Staying Sickness*, University of Arizona Press, Tucson, 1974.

76. D. M. Bahr and J. R. Haefer, Song in Piman curing, *Ethnomusicology* 22:89–122, 1978.
77. M. U. Everett, *White Mountain Apache Health and Illness: An Ethnographic Study of Medical Decision Making*, University of Arizona, Tucson, 1971.
78. T. H. Lewis, An Indian healer's preventive medicine procedure, *Hospital and Community Psychiatry* 25:94–95, 1974.
79. C. Acosta, Zuni healing societies: The clown fraternity, in: *The Healing Community* (R. Almond, ed.), Jason Aronson, New York, 1969.
80. S. M. Camazine, Traditional and Western health care among the Zuni Indians of New Mexico, *Social Science and Medicine, Part B, Medical Anthropology*. 14B:73–80, 1980.
81. R. M. Wagner, Peyotism, traditional religion and modern medicine: Changing healing traditions in the border areas, *Modern Medicine and Medical Anthropology in the U.S.-Mexico Border Populations*, Pan American Health Organization, Washington, D.C., 1978.
82. D. Dolan, *Summary Notes from the Rural Mental Health Workshop*, Washington State University, Pullman, 1973.
83. T. H. Lewis, A syndrome of depression and mutism in the Oglala Sioux, *American Journal of Psychiatry* 13:7, 1975.
84. J. Shore, American Indian suicide: Fact and fantasy, *Psychiatry* 38:86–91, 1975.
85. E. M. Pattison, Exorcism and psychotherapy: A case of collaboration, in: *Religious Systems and Psychotherapy* (R. H. Cox, ed.), Charles C Thomas, Springfield, Illinois, 1973.

Index

GPSR Compliance

The European Union's (EU) General Product Safety Regulation (GPSR) is a set of rules that requires consumer products to be safe and our obligations to ensure this.

If you have any concerns about our products, you can contact us on ProductSafety@springernature.com

In case Publisher is established outside the EU, the EU authorized representative is:

Springer Nature Customer Service Center GmbH
Europaplatz 3
69115 Heidelberg, Germany

Batch number: 10854096

Printed by Printforce, the Netherlands